TRANSFORMING CLINICAL PRACTICE USING THE MINDBODY APPROACH

TRANSFORMING CLINICAL PRACTICE USING THE MINDBODY APPROACH
A Radical Integration

Editor

Brian Broom

Sub-editor

Peta Joyce

Routledge
Taylor & Francis Group

LONDON AND NEW YORK

First published 2013 by Karnac Books Ltd.

Published 2018 by Routledge
2 Park Square, Milton Park, Abingdon, Oxon OX14 4RN
711 Third Avenue, New York, NY 10017, USA

Routledge is an imprint of the Taylor & Francis Group, an informa business

British Library Cataloguing in Publication Data

A C.I.P. for this book is available from the British Library

ISBN-13: 9781780490618 (pbk)

Typeset by V Publishing Solutions Pvt Ltd., Chennai, India

CONTENTS

ACKNOWLEDGEMENTS

This book is about how healthcare can be transformed. It would not have been possible without the author-clinicians who have undergone the personal transformative processes necessary to be MindBody clinicians, and been willing to write about them. I am grateful for the almost unremitting goodwill from everyone, and especially for those who really wished they were doing other things more natural to them than writing for a fussy and occasionally intrusive editor. Certainly there is great variety in the approaches taken by the authors, but the genuineness and honesty that pervades this book is astonishing. Thank you, all of you.

Many of the authors have gone through the MindBody Healthcare post-graduate programme in the Department of Psychotherapy at AUT University, Auckland. Looking back on the last twelve years I am very grateful for the support provided by the University for setting up the programme. Dr Peter Greener, then Head of the School for Public Health and Psychosocial Studies, persuaded the University to take the risk. The Dean, Professor Max Abbott, accepted the risk. Peter Greener's successor, Professor Janis Paterson, has been equally supportive. Margot Solomon and Josie Goulding (also a co-leader of the programme), as Heads of the Department of Psychotherapy, have been staunchly positive, committed and supportive. In particular, Josie, apart from her invaluable co-leadership, has carried much of the administrative end of the programme, and her presence and knowledge of how the University system works have made the course viable, and mitigated the potential loneliness inherent in a pioneering program which, initially, few people understood.

Our sincere thanks must go to all the patients and clients whose stories have contributed to this book. All these stories have been altered in name and certain details to ensure that no one is identifiable.

I cannot over-emphasize my gratitude to Peta Joyce who at an early stage volunteered to act as coordinator of the book drafts, and as a reviewer of the technical aspects of the writing, though her role expanded beyond this into some aspects of content. She marshalled everybody very gently, and attended to the many details that emerge when one is managing eighteen authors. Peta kept on saying she was enjoying herself, a testimony to an indomitable spirit, which is also in evidence in her chapter contribution written from the perspective of a patient. She is also a clinician who has been through the AUT MindBody programme. My sincere thanks to her husband Don who eagle-eyed the references. That was a task to put me off even attempting this project!

My sincere thanks go to Oliver Rathbone and his staff at Karnac Books. The project had to be delayed because of serious illness in my family, and they have been nothing but understanding and gracious.

Finally, to Alison, my wife, I wish to express my gratitude for her decades-long loving support and interest. If it were not for her and her attitudes, it would have been impossible for us to have negotiated as well as we have the unexpected complexities of our lives since we moved to Auckland in 2008; and certainly impossible to see another book on MindBody matters published.

CONTRIBUTORS

Brian Broom, MB ChB, FRACP, MSc (Immunology), MNZAP, is a consultant immunologist at Auckland City Hospital. He is also a registered psychotherapist. He initiated MindBody Healthcare post-graduate training in the department of psychotherapy at AUT University, and co-leads the programme. His other books are *Somatic Illness and the Patient's Other Story* (1997) and *Meaning-Full Disease. How personal experience and meanings initiate and maintain physical illness* (2007). His special interests are MindBody psychotherapy treatments of physical disease, the development of MindBody theory, and the evolution of MindBody educational and research approaches.

Sharon Carey, BSc (Hons), NZRD, PGCertHSc (MindBody Healthcare) is a specialist dietitian for allergy and clinical immunology at Auckland City Hospital, and takes a MindBody approach to people with chronic conditions such as food hypersensitivity, irritable bowel syndrome and obesity. She was awarded the *Cow & Gate Prize for Nutrition* with her degree in Applied Human Nutrition (Dietetics) at the University of Wales Institute, Cardiff. She has qualifications in NZ dietetics and sports nutrition.

Chris Cornelius (pseudonym) is an academic social scientist and health services researcher employed by a large university.

Marlies Dorrestein, Dip OT, PGCert (Occupational Practice), DipCounselling, is a lecturer in the Department of Occupational Science and Therapy at AUT University, Auckland. She trained originally in occupational therapy in Liverpool, and is currently completing a Masters degree in MindBody Healthcare. Her special interest is the benefit of contemplative (e.g. mindfulness) practice alongside occupational practice for educators, students and healthcare practitioners, as part of a MindBody approach in tertiary education and healthcare.

Yvonne Evans, TTC, Dip Tchg, H Dip Tchg, Adv Dip Tchg, M Counselling, PGCertHSc (MindBody Healthcare), works as a guidance counsellor in a rural high school using a MindBody—Narrative Therapy approach. She worked for thirty years as a primary teacher, including fourteen years as the principal of a special school. Her publications include articles on children's stress management, counsellor care, and the experience of undertaking research.

Leeanne Ford, Dip HSc RN, PGDipHSc (MindBody Healthcare) is a registered nurse currently working in the hospice environment. She is passionate about the practice of mindfulness and its role in integrating a MindBody approach within her work.

Josie Goulding, Dip Psychotherapy, Dip Nursing, PGDip Sexual Health Counselling, MHSc (Hon), MNZAP is a registered psychotherapist and head of the department of psychotherapy at AUT University, Auckland. She teaches on the MindBody Programme and has a small private psychotherapy practice. Her special areas of interest are psychotherapy, gender and sexuality, and MindBody matters as they present for both the client and therapist. Her masters' thesis completed in 2003 was entitled *Embodied relationships: the therapist's experience*.

Emma Harris, BA, Grad Dip Psych Soc, MHSc (Psychotherapy), PGDipHSc (MindBody Healthcare), is a psychotherapist in private practice in Auckland. Her passions include working with each person's unique presentation, improving peoples' health outcomes in her local community, and facilitating the integration of MindBody ideas into mainstream medical healthcare.

Chris Hayes, B Med (Hons), FANZCA, FFPMANZCA, M Med (Pain Management) is a pain medicine specialist working in the public system at John Hunter Hospital, Newcastle, Australia. He has been director of the Hunter Integrated Pain Service since its foundation in 1997 after initially training in anaesthetics. His research interests are based on a "whole person" approach to pain which includes MindBody, nutritional and lifestyle components. Pain education is a major focus and relevant information is available on www.hnehealth.nsw.gov.au/pain.

Paul Hemmingsen, BSc (Hons), PGDipHSc (MindBody Healthcare), ANZAP Dip. Adult Psychotherapy, NZAP Adv. Clin. Practice, is a registered psychotherapist working with the Student Health Service at the University of Otago, and in private practice. After a career in microbiology and dairy farming, he began training in psychotherapy some twenty years ago, gaining a diploma in self psychology. His recent passion for MindBody healthcare has enhanced his capacity to understand and work with his diverse range of clients. He enjoys working alongside general medical practitioners and helping them with their difficult case presentations.

Peta Joyce, BA, Dip Holistic Pulsing, PGCertHSc (MindBody Healthcare) completed her MindBody training in 2008. She has extensive experience in integrative and body-focussed counselling and therapy, mentoring and supervision and group facilitation. She is in private practice in Auckland as a supervisor and MindBody therapist, teaches at Wellpark College of Natural Therapies, and trains people to supervise in the health, not-for-profit and community sectors.

Karen Lindsay, MBChB, BSc (Biomed Sci), MRCP, a United Kingdom—trained rheumatologist, moved to New Zealand in 2009, and now works as a rheumatologist and immunology research fellow at Auckland City Hospital. Her special interests are MindBody approaches to auto-immune disorders including inflammatory eye disease, and using qualitative research methods to explore the effects of the MindBody approach on patients and clinicians.

Susan Lugton, Dip Phty, PGDip Phty (manips), PGCertHSc (acupuncture) is a musculoskeletal physiotherapist with post-graduate training in manipulative physiotherapy, breathing rehabilitation and MindBody healthcare. She has a passion for the MindBody approach within the physiotherapy healthcare model. Her clinic, *Moving Well*, in Auckland (since 2000) specializes in the treatment of headaches, neck and chronic body pain, breathing disorders and conditions such as endometriosis, chronic fatigue and irritable bowel. She teaches breathing awareness and self-nurture strategies at hospice groups and the Encore cancer programme.

Mark Murphy, BA (Hons), MA, PG Dip Discursive Therapies, PGCertHSc (MindBody Healthcare), Dip gestalt Psychotherapy, is a registered psychotherapist in private practice, a lecturer in counselling studies at Vision College, both in Christchurch, and a trainer with the Gestalt Institute of New Zealand. His professional interests include contemporary gestalt therapy, working with men in psychotherapy and with people suffering from physical illness related to life stress and distress. His other interests include poetry, art, the cosmos, blackberry grubbing, and yoga.

Stephanie Oak, BA (Hons), BMed (Hons), FRANZCP, FFPMANZCA, is a consultant psychiatrist and pain medicine specialist in the public health system at John Hunter Hospital, Newcastle, Australia. She is Head of Department, Consultation Liaison Psychiatry and has been working with the Hunter Integrated Pain Service for the past 14 years.

Renske van den Brink, MBChB, DipObs, FRNZCGP, DipCounselling, PGDipHSc (MindBody Healthcare), is a general medical practitioner and counsellor . After 10 years in general practice in Auckland, she completed a Diploma of Psychosynthesis Counselling in 2002. She now works in private practice specializing in supporting people to explore the emotional aspects of their physical symptoms. She is a part-time senior teaching fellow in the Department of General Practice at Auckland University, teaching patient-centred communication skills, and does similar work as a partner in her private company called Connect Communications.

Iona Winter, PGDipSocial Practice, PGCertHSc (MindBody Healthcare), GradDip Psychotherapy, MNZAP, is a registered psychotherapist in private practice. For twenty years she has provided counselling, psychotherapy, supervision and facilitation to individuals and groups. Iona works holistically, exploring the interconnectedness of mind, body and spirit. Having bi-cultural whakapapa (ancestry) her practice embodies the land, Aotearoa (New Zealand), on which she resides. Iona is currently working on a novel.

Sharon Wood, BHS, CNMT, Dip Mass, PGCertHSc (MindBody Healthcare), has been actively involved in private practice massage therapy and therapist education for the past eighteen years. Over the past decade she has actively researched, written and presented on stress, and, in particular, the healing dimensions that touch and massage can offer.

CHAPTER ONE

Introduction: transforming clinical practice using the MindBody approach

Brian Broom

The extraordinary stories that appear in this book provide unique, multi-faceted, and rich perspectives on what happens when ordinary clinicians become MindBody clinicians; committed to non-dualistic, whole person healthcare. The result is transformation; and this process begins in the clinician. Personal hurdles and blockages are faced and surmounted, particularly those concerning emotion, self-belief, and styles of intimate relating. The clinician's attitudes and ways of functioning with patients are both subtly and radically transformed, nervously at first, but then confidently and often thrillingly in the end. Patients, previously stuck and chronically ill with various conditions, frequently get better; the patient is transformed. In many cases, this transformation flows through the clinicians' workplace, as colleagues, often initially sceptical and resistant, see the clinical results for themselves. This book is therefore about a kind of transformation that ripples through established systems, a person-to-person grass-roots movement potentially involving all players and all structures.

The origins of MindBody Healthcare

Some background is needed to explain how MindBody Healthcare arose in New Zealand. Back in 1980, I was a young consultant physician at the Christchurch School of Medicine. I had previously trained as a clinical immunologist in Birmingham, London and Montreal under the generous auspices of the (then) New Zealand Medical Research Council. In 1976, I returned to Christchurch to set up a clinical and research immunology group. Five years into this burgeoning career process, I was questioning whether I could survive another thirty years or so of increasingly laboratory-oriented medicine. I was very frustrated with my occupational drift away from people towards mechanism, and desired more engagement with the psychological, philosophical, and spiritual aspects of healthcare; or more broadly, the role of human subjectivity in disease.

So, in a classic midlife crisis, I resigned my career in academic clinical immunology and started training in psychiatry. I really had only vague ideas as to where this might lead me, and the ensuing long periods of confusion and uncertainty were difficult to manage emotionally. I had a young family, felt isolated and alienated from my erstwhile internal medicine colleagues and peers, and did not feel particularly comfortable with merely shifting from internal medicine to psychiatry. My interest and general orientation had always been towards integration and synthesis, with a focus on people and their lives especially in relation to illness and disease. Simply moving from a mind-neglecting specialty to a body-neglecting specialty was ultimately not going to warrant the enormous upheaval I was visiting upon myself.

Behind all this was the propulsive idea that somehow mind, body, and spirit were not separate compartments, but day-to-day living dimensions of the person that needed to be viewed as a whole for the best care of that person's suffering and trajectory towards healing. I certainly had a body orientation from my internal medicine background, and though in reality I did not know a lot about healthy bodies I had a reasonable grip on bodily disease as seen through the dualistic and reductive lens of orthodox biomedicine. As time went by, whilst getting experience in psychiatry, I became increasingly fascinated with the psyche. Eventually, I became a psychotherapist trained in the psychodynamic tradition, with a particular emphasis upon interpersonal, relational, self psychological, and object relations approaches. Last, but not least, there was my upbringing in an intense form of conservative Protestantism which drove a search to make sense of spirituality in the modern world. Given my integrative and synthesizing proclivities, I found it impossible to take the usual reductive options, to either deny spirituality altogether, or simply settle for a spirituality kept neatly separate from the stimulating and challenging data emerging from the natural and social sciences; and separate from any serious grappling with the meaning of illness and suffering.

In 1987, I returned to immunology practice, combining it with psychotherapy practice, within the Arahura Centre in Christchurch, New Zealand, as one of a group of people intent on integrating all elements of personhood into healthcare practice. This story has been alluded to elsewhere (Broom, 1997; Broom, 2007), but there is one aspect that needs emphasizing. As I began combining clinical immunology and psychotherapy practices, I was shaken by the constant appearance in patients of very physical disorders with life stories to match. These stories seemed to explain why these patients were ill, and working with them in the clinical setting seemed to be very relevant to why they got better. I started to see that many diseases were full of meaning (Broom, 2007), even reaching the intensity of somatic metaphor (Broom, 2002), where the physical representation of disease in the body seems to communicate the same meanings that are being expressed by the patient in words. For instance, the patient who presented with a severe facial rash and who repeatedly declared she is "keeping a brave face" on her husband's depression.

These phenomena began to affect the way I practised. They stimulated a different kind of clinical approach to patients, whereby the stories and meaningful elements were attended to as an extension of orthodox healthcare practice. Initially, my focus was the patient's "other" story (Broom, 1997) and particularly personal meaning and its relations to illness (Broom, 2002; Broom, 2007). Inevitably, this led to a much larger journey of exploration of the paradigmatic assumptions underpinning medical practice and notions of healing, as well as to the development of clinical skills (Broom, 1997; Broom, 2000) necessary for clinicians if they were going to be able to attend to both the physicality and the subjectivity of their patients, which I was now seeing as crucial to optimum healing outcomes.

Gradually, people became interested in what I was doing, and over the next two decades I supervised many clinicians, and actively taught the story and meanings approach to illness in many seminars, workshops, and lectures both in New Zealand and internationally. It became clear that unless such clinicians were accompanied, supervised, educated, supported, and held over a sustained period, it was very difficult for them to enact the changes needed in their clinical workplaces. As we will see in the chapters that follow, changing from a limited reductionist biomedical or dualistic approach is very difficult for many clinicians, especially initially. The challenges faced are configured by many things, including each individual's emotional makeup, and by the inertia and constraints (some of them imagined rather than real) of the healthcare system they work in.

A training programme was needed. Initial attempts to get this established at the Christchurch School of Medicine, supported by the Dean of the School at that time, failed because academic departments in the School would not support the venture. The reported reasons were diverse. In the case of Internal Medicine the problem seemed to be mystification as to what we were trying to do. In the case of General Practice the reason appeared to be a fear of being viewed as scientifically lightweight. In the case of Psychiatry the problem seemed to be a rather rigid and unimaginative construction of what psychiatry should allow, or be involved in.

The project lost momentum for several years, but revived again when Dr Peter Greener (Head of the School of Public Health and Psychosocial Studies, at the AUT University in Auckland) and I started discussions regarding the establishment of a training programme within the Department of Psychotherapy. The University needed to be convinced. Four years later, in 2006, we enrolled nineteen MindBody Healthcare students into a part-time multidisciplinary post-graduate Certificate, Diploma and Masters programme; the MindBody papers of which are conducted over two years. The other side of this story is that in the clinical professions there are many clinicians who want to transform their practices to become more whole person-oriented.

The clinical and theoretical substance of the MindBody Healthcare approach to clinical work has been systematically detailed elsewhere (Broom, 1991; Broom, 1997; Broom, 2000; Broom, 2002; Broom, 2007; Broom, 2010; Broom, Booth and Schubert, 2012), and will be further explicated, coloured and nuanced by all the authors that follow, as they speak from their own personal experiences of transformation.

To orientate readers from the outset, I will provide a short summary of the scope and methodology of the MindBody approach.

The MindBody approach: some general comments

The context is that of an ordinary clinician in an ordinary clinical setting, whether that be in medicine, nursing, physiotherapy, occupational therapy, dietetics, psychotherapy or any other discipline. Most of these disciplines have developed out of a dualistic model of the person, and more recently have become hostage to a narrow scientific, evidence-based medicine; almost entirely based on the treatment of groups of patients rather than individual persons (Broom, 1997).

Let us briefly touch on the place of biomedicine in the MindBody approach. The latter encompasses modern biomedical evidence-based practice, but broadens a clinician's view of disease and patient care well beyond normative biomedical perspectives. It values much of biomedicine, and assumes that diagnosis and useful orthodox biomedical interventions will be utilized where appropriate (Broom, 1997). Nevertheless, in many cases, deploying the MindBody approach may actually mean that biomedical interventions are not needed.

What makes the MindBody approach so different to biomedicine is the emphasis it places on subjectivity (of both the clinician and the patient), on relationships (especially between the clinician and the patient), and on the intimate relations between life experience and the development and perpetuation of illness. The patient's story, and the meanings heard and held in the clinical space, are seen as crucial to the healing process. Thus, from this perspective, the group data approach of evidence-based medicine is deeply flawed because of the way it makes individual patient stories invisible. Critically, the MindBody clinician can hold both the ordinary biomedical approach and the MindBody approach together as part of a greater therapeutic whole.

The meaning of illness is important to the MindBody approach, and for me arose from what I was seeing clinically in my work with patients, as both a physician and a psychotherapist. When my (then) new colleague and friend Michael Harlow pointed me to Georg Groddeck's early twentieth century volume, *The Meaning of Illness* (Groddeck, 1928), very late in the writing of my first book, I was both delighted and deeply reassured to find that Groddeck had seen the same relations between disease and life meanings; the same kind of stories. Then, later again, I was to chance upon Luis Chiozza's writings (Chiozza, 1998a; Chiozza, 1998b), finally translated from Spanish and supporting the reality of symbolic illness, albeit from a rather forced psychoanalytic perspective. Of course the discourse of symbolic illness has many more roots and sources (Broom, Booth and Schubert, 2012) than can be addressed in this introductory chapter.

There are many other aspects to the MindBody approach, and over its evolution there have been both general and very specific contributions from many sources, much of it by accretion or osmosis. It is difficult to honour all of these adequately. My psychotherapy interests are eclectic. Brought up to see in what way other people were wrong, I have learned that just about every school of thought, clinical framework, or theory has some value and some contribution to whole person medicine, mainly because they all reflect amplification of some aspect of personhood that the originator of the idea or theory was particularly drawn to. I have been drawn to aspects of many traditions, but feel no need to find safe harbour within any one of them.

Yet again, some aspects of the MindBody approach were crystallised in eureka moments, notably when confronted in a clinical setting with an extraordinary conjunction between disease phenomenology and the patient's personal meanings that could not be explained using biomedical reductive theory. I can remember very distinctive clinical moments of hearing such stories, which stimulated goose bumps and tingling up my spine, and which pushed me over yet another threshold into new territory regarding mind and body relationships.

In my earlier books the meaning of illness and the patient's story were, together, my portals of entry to a whole person approach, and the organizing concepts for my explorations and practice with patients. They are easily presented in time-constrained consultations, and intuitively comprehended by patients. From the beginning, these focussing concepts arose not only from the language of patients as they talked spontaneously about their lives and their illnesses, but also germinated within a field of ideas, theories, and certain schools of clinical practice and philosophical thought. Thus the MindBody approach represents many sources, and honours the rich multidimensionality of persons, existence, relationships, and the world; just about everything is a potential source. There are both general sources and very specific sources and I will now summarize these.

The nature of the MindBody approach

The mindbody clinician fosters a relational clinical space or "clearing" (Heidegger, 1935; Heidegger, 1962) where that which needs to emerge for healing can do so. In this clinical space both protagonists are primarily human beings-in-the-world, albeit with the secondary and contextual roles of clinician and patient. The clinician respectfully invites the patient to be fully present, creating a setting that both allows for it and insists on it (Broom, 1991). Crucially, this presence includes not just the patient's symptoms (with a view to diagnosis and biomedical treatment) but also their story (Broom, 1991), feelings, and potentially any or all of the relational elements usually rendered invisible (Merleau-Ponty, 1969) by normative clinical processes. The clinician, in turn, is fully present for the patient, drawing on their own feelings and embodied awareness to make sense of the patient's needs. This sounds immense, even impossible, but in reality the story is in the minor (sic) elements that are "always already symbolically mediated" (Ricoeur, 1984); if we use our senses to see what is present on the margins of our awareness. The two people are certainly separate but the relational dynamic is intimate, trusting, and determinedly authentic (Levenson, 1974).

The process of story-sharing by the patient, heard and responded to by the clinician, is based on warm, active listening, and a determination to hear the patient's usually invisible subjective experience. The clinical attitudes and skills deployed in this process are derived from Carl Roger's client-centred therapy, psychodynamic and psychoanalytical therapies, and the phenomenological philosophies. In accordance with modern affect and attachment theory, and all schools of psychotherapy, the clinician accepts that affect, emotion, and feelings, have a major role in the process (Broom, Booth and Schubert, 2012). These happen as part of the consultation and must be noticed, responded to, named, amplified, contained, and warmly accompanied. Many clinicians need practice to develop these skills, because biomedical training tends to constrain or stifle emotion.

As this process is enacted, the body-only, biomedical history (with which the patient usually presents) must be integrated with the other story (Broom, 1997) which emerges (Broom, Booth and Schubert, 2012) between the clinician and the patient. Often this other story is simply captured in a pattern of meaning(s) (Broom, 2007), and opens out into the therapeutic clearing in a way that is easy for both parties to grasp, and then use in the forward movement of the treatment. Sometimes the disease turns out to be so clearly and obviously full of meaning that we can call it a somatic metaphor or symbolic disorder (Groddeck, 1928; Chiozza, 1998a; Chiozza, 1998b; Broom, 2002; Broom, 2007).

The fundamental premise in all of this is that meanings, relational dynamics, and other dimensions of subjectivity do play a role in the development and perpetuation of disease. Attending to these can play a powerful role in the healing process.

A bigger story, integrating the biomedical narrative and the other story, is allowed to develop by both parties. This is enabled by various means, including clinical tentativeness and sensitivity, the clinician's ability to explain non-dual ways of seeing illness, and of course helped by the patient's desperation (Broom, 1997). In reality many patients know that they and their diseases encompass much more than that which is usually allowed or is visible in the orthodox clinical consultation. If the MindBody approach is enacted skilfully and compassionately, many patients will allow an integration of their physical manifestations and their life experience, and agree to a tentative or determined exploration, to help resolve pathogenic story elements.

Informed by object relations theory, this exploration involves a high quality, empathic and committed accompanying of the patient by the clinician. There is a clear intention to call the patient forth (Levinas, 1996), and, according to self psychology concepts, to evoke the patient's agency and emotional mobility. There is a clear valuing of the patient's strengths, as well as gentle handling of vulnerabilities, along with attention to family and cultural elements and the relationships between social networks and illness (Antonovsky, 1979; Antonovsky, 1987; Antonovsky, 1996).

The general intent is for the patient to have an experience of warmth, empathy, and understanding; as well as having their disorder viewed through multi-factorial and multi-dimensional perspectives (in which physical, subjective, and systems elements are seamlessly interwoven). The therapist is person-centred, not theory-centred. Whilst all the theories and perspectives mentioned in the above paragraphs have informed the development of ideas of personhood underpinning the MindBody approach, when it comes to the clinical encounter the clinician meets each patient as a unique person, the only person ever to tell this particular story. In a sense, the clinician comes to each patient afresh, with no assumptions as to what an illness may mean.

In short, the clinician's models of personhood and disease are more unitary than dualistic. He is both person-centred and disease-centred. The meanings of illness are actively sought, and the patient is seen as expressing themself in multiple dimensions simultaneously; all of which are potential access points for healing. Great store is put on the therapeutic value of skilful holding of the patient's vulnerability and need to be heard and understood within the clinical relationship.

While much of the MindBody approach is rooted in principles derived from psychotherapy, it is important to note that many MindBody clinicians are not psychotherapists, as will become evident in the following chapters. Any clinician with the intention, and good relational capacity, can become MindBody-oriented and accomplished in their own discipline. In fact it transpires that psychotherapists have as much to learn as non-psychotherapists when training to do this work. MindBody clinicians need not be super-human, and many do not have the time or capacity to do all that is needed on their own. Thus, shared care between MindBody clinicians from different disciplines is desirable.

Why "MindBody"?

What about the term MindBody itself? There is no satisfactory labelling or categorization for this approach without becoming reductionist. We have used "story", "whole person", "the meaning of illness", "meaning-full disease", and MindBody as useful and somewhat interchangeable indicators of our emphases; but they all fall short in some way, failing to express the entirety of what we are doing. In the end, we have resorted to calling it the MindBody approach, which for us encompasses body, physicality, subjectivity, relationship, family, culture, spirituality, or whatever emerges when personal meanings and stories are allowed into the clinical encounter and understood to play a crucial role in the development and perpetuation of human illness and disease.

We might well have continued to call it the "Story approach", because patient and clinician stories are right at the centre of the work, but the term MindBody seemed more acceptable when it came to proposing a post-graduate University programme. Some might wonder if we are just replicating the emphasis of Mind/Body Medicine, which commonly seems to be a mix of orthodox medicine plus alternative therapies and some psychological elements. At the heart of the MindBody approach is a more radical non-dualistic personhood, in which meaning and subjectivity are as crucial as organs and physicality. This determination to attend to both subjectivity and physicality is applicable to every form of medicine or healing.

Finally, some might ask why not the "Psychosomatic approach"? The answer is that the term psychosomatic carries far too many residues of mind and body dualism and linear mind-to-body causation. For instance, its largely dualistic assumptions do not allow it to embrace many of the so-called organic diseases treated by internal medicine physicians. In contrast, from a unitary MindBody perspective we consider personal stories to be potentially relevant in all disease (Broom, Booth and Schubert, 2012).

The training of MindBody clinicians

The real story of this book lies in what really happens to clinicians who undergo MindBody training, who undertake the change from a biomedical modelling to whole person modelling of illness and practice, and then what happens to their patients.

The AUT University post-graduate MindBody Healthcare programme teaching experience will be discussed by Josie Goulding (Chapter Seventeen), who co-leads the programme. She provides insights into the ways students struggle with dualism, and their gradual movement towards competency in whole person healthcare. It becomes clear that this process frequently involves intense personal dilemmas and crises.

The training provides a theoretical, philosophical, and scientific framework, to enable clinicians to feel both legitimate and comfortable when working with their patients as whole persons, in a non-dualistic way (in contrast with the almost universal dualistic mind or body way of orthodox medical and other allied medical healthcare practices). This is a process that takes a lot of time, discussion and excavation, because dualistic thinking is so entrenched in Western healthcare and clinical thinking and practice. Moreover, the programme seeks to model and coach the skills needed for clinicians to both remain competent in an orthodox sense and still work with patients as whole persons, the MindBody, in their normal clinical time-space.

These things are easily stated, but they are difficult for the students to achieve because of restraints imposed by conventional scopes of practice, time and collegial pressures, supposed patient expectations, various imagined fears and difficulties, and the sense of isolation that develops when one starts to become different. Sustained support, encouragement, modelling and supervision over the two years of the programme all help with these issues. Without exception, a certain amount of tumult develops for each clinician student. Fear, uncertainty, and disorientation, are normally experienced in the first few weeks and months, only to be gradually replaced by a sense of enlargement, by the thrill of discovering a new clinical panorama, and a growing competence in actually being able to see and respond to the previously invisible patient stories that are relevant to their illness presentation. It is remarkable to observe the students moving from clumsy, fearful, and trembling beginnings, to being confident MindBody clinicians able to function skilfully in their clinical settings. They become able to articulate clearly to both patients and colleagues what they are doing in their own disciplinary version of a whole person approach, and why they are doing it.

Essentially the transformation is a growth movement by the clinician. The objective is a confident and competent ability to help patients and clients see that their illnesses and their lives are interwoven in a way that makes it necessary to address both. That is, the clinician can integrate, with some degree of comfort, both subjectivity (mind) and physicality (body) aspects of the suffering person's human story in the same clinical time/space. Whilst the training certainly involves growth in both conceptual understanding of MindBody healing processes and then the requisite clinical skills, it all turns out to be much more than this. I suspect readers will be jolted by some of the personal material that comes into view. We are talking about a kind of healthcare and medicine that calls forth a review of story and a movement to health in both the clinician and the patient.

Virtually without exception, by the end of the two years, each student has grown dramatically in their own way and according to their own discipline, and these changes are full of drama. It is really important to note that all these students came into the programme as mature clinicians, apparently firmly (if not satisfyingly) ensconced in their respective healthcare professions. The majority had been on some kind of sustained personal and, in some cases, difficult searches for a new form of clinical practice. Most have been impelled forward by a realization that there must be another way; something more to healing practice than that which they have received either by training, through personal experience, or by edict of institutional or professional scopes of practice.

This desire for a different kind of practice has been stimulated by a variety of factors. There is the very common experience of the barrenness of clinical practice rooted in mechanistic and physicalist assumptions. Some of the authors have personal experience of the failure of such models to reach and respond to their own suffering. Others are driven by a general intuitive sense that there is much more to the healing response to human persons than is generally considered or indeed allowed by the particular system in which the practitioner has emerged. Others simply feel that there is something wrong in the way we practice, but which is hard to articulate or conceptualize. Then there are those who have observed in their own life or in a patient's story that contrary to any model provided within their orthodox disciplinary setting, some life event has been closely connected with the onset and development of a physical illness that could not be construed as merely psychosomatic.

A darker side to modern medicine

In short, there is a shadow side to modern medicine and healthcare. I suggest that it boils down to this; that there is something profoundly disrespectful of human personhood in how Western healthcare is practised. This arises from the dualistic view of the nature of persons, and results in a neglecting of the relations between illness and disease and the subjectivity aspects of the whole person, which include stories, life events, relationships, and meanings.

On the surface, the idea that we can indeed transform current clinical practice might suggest more than a whiff of arrogance, presumption, or idealism. In this book, we, as a collective of authors, risk that judgment, and contest it anyway. The changes undergone by these clinicians, and documented here, are urgently needed on a wider scale. Why on earth do we attempt something so big? Or, perhaps, what draws some of us to tip the world we know upside down? Whether it is our own world or that of our patients, these worlds are long established, have many merits, are heavy with inertia, and are rich with personal, familial, and cultural history.

Ironically, I began to write this introduction in the shadow of an arch-idealist. I was sitting under a tree in St Francis' country, rural Italy, six kilometres from Assisi, as the sun started at last to lose its strength, modestly assisted by a strengthening breeze. A rooster crowed constantly just beyond the vegetable garden. Listening intently, I could hear distant dogs barking in every direction. Larks and swifts swooped above me. A wafting smell of cow dung triggered a memory of standing by my mother as she hand-milked the family Friesian, and squirted a stream of warm milk towards me. Before me was a glowing reddish-yellow wheat field, confined by deep green boundary-riding oaks and ilex, and shouldered by a field of ancient centrally-pruned olive trees underpinned by black, ring-like shadows. Around me there was a clutter of sheds and machinery, grey faded hay bales, scattered ceramic pots with lemon trees, basil, and geraniums. In short, a kind of Arcadian-Italian version of the seemingly endless hot summer days of my New Zealand childhood, the dessicating "nor-westers" sweeping across the Canterbury Plains from the Southern Alps, the dry rank smells of the chicken house, the tail of the cow lazily flicking away flies, and the cheerful yellows of flowering broom.

I was staying in a house with fifty centimetre stone walls, floor tiles trodden smooth, and window shutters of thick oak, all pointing to some kind of permanence. Down the road, in Assisi, the same stone sustains astonishing monuments to human engineering, architectural imagination and creativity, housing many vivid treasures, symbols of both desire and the discipline of desire. The frescoes in the magnificent upper and lower churches of the Basilica map the story of St. Francis, a supreme idealist; aspiring to poverty, chastity, and obedience. The richness and complexity of human endeavour, aspiration, paradox, contradiction and irony openly intermingle. The well-equipped visitor with a digital camera, and every contrivance to make travel manageable, stands shoulder-to-shoulder with an earnest Franciscan brother limited to wearing cloak, breeches, and girdle (Hay, 1964).

While I was in Italy, the northern region was hit by earthquakes, and back in Christchurch, Canterbury, New Zealand, aftershocks from the devastating February 2011 earthquake were still terrifying the populace. In Assisi itself, the architectural monuments showed ample evidence of restoration from the 1997 earthquake. Reflecting on this, I found myself drawing parallels with the ways in which the magnificent edifice of Western healthcare, built upon biomedical foundations, is shaking.

Health economics evidence suggests that on current projections the cost of healthcare, largely driven by technological advance and medical opportunity, is going to become unsupportable, with grave consequences for the social fabric. Public health and epidemiological data suggest that a major determinant of health is a person's social network and support, and occupational meaning and satisfaction. Illness and disease should no longer be construed as merely a breakdown in bodily machinery, and proper health provision is no longer a hoped for technological rectification of an isolatable biochemical dysfunction. The burgeoning epidemic of obesity, diabetes, and other life-style diseases suggest the powerful influence of socio-cultural issues in ill health, and that the narrow seeking for biomedical answers is a kind of physico-materialist craziness. Many patients are tired of the common healthcare clinical pattern, of being passed from one organ specialist to another with little communication between them, and little interest by each specialist in any aspect of the person except the specialist's own particular organ system. Many patients do not feel listened to.

This is the century of chronic conditions. Whilst biomedicine has been very effective with infectious disease and acute conditions, chronic conditions are more resistant to biomedical modelling and therapies. It is around chronic conditions that the health crisis is largely arising, at least in the developed nations. The MindBody approach does not eschew a role for biomedical therapies as one dimension of treating the whole, and undoubtedly biomedicine will remain an important player in chronic diseases. But there is a sickness inside the basilica of modern healthcare. On the whole, biomedicine fails to comprehend that it is the whole person who is sick, not just this organ or that body system. This is what the MindBody approach addresses. The message from this book is that a healthcare practice that limits itself to the body is always going to be profoundly inadequate, and this is particularly relevant in chronic conditions. The fundamental message is that all kinds of clinician can adopt a MindBody approach in their own disciplines.

No matter how advanced our biomedical care has become, there are shifts coming in healthcare, and such shifts must include MindBody integration in all health conditions. This volume illustrates what that can look like. We do not imitate St. Francis and disavow (in our case) the whole biomedical edifice. Neither can we sit comfortably in our professional landscapes, enjoying the ambience, and do nothing about the person-denying assumptions and behaviours of modern healthcare. We want to show that the ordinary clinician can become an entirely different kind of clinician in whom the virtues of biomedicine can be enlarged into a really integrative whole person healing enterprise.

The MindBody clinician's story

In the MindBody approach we find that each patient has a unique story, which is often crucial to treatment. Likewise, here, we find that each clinician presents a story with unique elements, and, put together, they display what an integrated MindBody practice looks like from the inside. I did not ask the clinicians to contribute primarily because they were writers, but because they were doing or had done the work to become person-centred clinicians. The styles of writing and routes towards transformation differ as much as people always differ, but when combined, we see the extensive reach of healthcare based on a MindBody approach. Whilst this book is principally about clinician transformation, it also includes chapters written by two thoughtful patients who have found healing through the MindBody approach, and a chapter written by the lead clinicians of an Australian Pain Medicine clinical service who have adopted the approach as their undergirding clinical philosophy.

Sharon Carey (Chapter two), a nutritionist, captures how patients can feel when not considered from a whole person perspective. It is sobering to see that biomedical modelling of physical illnesses may lead to a perpetuation of patients' symptoms and suffering. More than that, it shows that a clinician's frustration, disenchantment, and struggle with the chronicity and ineffectiveness arising from such modelling can lead to the clinician becoming ill too. It is obvious that some clinicians (and some disciplines such as surgery) fit the reductive biomedical paradigm better than others. Carey's story shows that there is something deadening about the way the biomedical model configures most clinical practice. And it demonstrates the sense of relief and liberation for some young clinicians when they discover whole person ways of approaching clinical problems.

Mark Murphy (Chapter three), a gestalt therapist, explores the nature of the intimate healing space that exists between and around two persons, drawing on Heidegger, Buber, Merleau Ponty and others. In this way he articulates our being-with patients and clients. Just as we get comfortable (or for practical non-theoretical souls, impatient) with this delicately nuanced conceptualization, he seamlessly models the gritty practical extension of this intimacy into the therapy room. The relational space is rich in its potential both for thought and for practice.

Paul Hemmingsen (Chapter four), a psychotherapist with the unlikely background of microbiology and dairy farming, takes the role of the therapist's body in the clinical space much further than most psychotherapists would ever contemplate. He has been forced by circumstances to overcome restrictive worldviews. He was attracted to MindBody training, but found himself unexpectedly and suddenly highly resistant to MindBody awareness. Curiosity and determination drove him to tackle his resistance. Allowing himself to encompass the body in the therapy context, he discovers that his own therapist body is an ongoing source of signalling regarding what is going on in the client. A kind of bodied conversation becomes a portal through which both he and the client pass to deal with traumatic life experiences and painful affects previously silenced or suppressed.

Emma Harris (Chapter five) is a non-medical psychotherapist. I am consistently struck by the power that the lay public and the mind-orientated professions have ceded to the biomedical disciplines, which, it seems, own the body. Harris, intent upon MindBody practice, initially finds it almost impossible to integrate the concepts, so strong are the roots of dualism and medical positivism in her life. She exposes the split between "being with", and "doing to" and shows that all clinicians, including psychotherapists, must learn to transcend these. In particular, psychotherapists need to challenge their implicit dualism, and must transform themselves to become fully embodied presences in the clinical space, creating a therapeutic space in which patient is free to integrate mind and body, and access healing. This is an important chapter for psychotherapists who have neglected the person as body, either by training, unconsciously-driven habit, or merely implicitly accepting the dualistic healthcare framework.

Renske van den Brink (Chapter six), a general medical practitioner and counsellor, also reveals the inside experience of the doctor confronted by the limitations of her profession, a journey triggered by her own illness, and the lack of clinical solutions for that illness. She stops looking outward, and begins a different internal journey resonant with the type of journey that all patients undertake when embarking on MindBody treatment. Along the way she reflects upon the implications of MindBody approaches for the conventional short consultation space provided by general practitioners. Deep listening is needed, and it does not need to be time-consuming. Much of what we should be hearing is already being revealed if only we would listen. Doctors listen to data that support pre-conceived patterns known as diagnoses; seemingly the rest is noise. Yet the noise carries magic for treatment and wellness. She tells of the "profoundly unsettling" call to shift from the certainties of diagnosis and "surrender to the chaos of the patient's immediate lived experience; allowing it to affect me and to influence me in the direction of where we go together." This is not one event but a growth process. It is not simply a fascination with the meaning of illness but also a journey into deep and intimate relationships with people.

Karen Lindsay (Chapter seven), a specialist physician in rheumatology working in a major metropolitan hospital, gives a vivid account of the personal and clinical chaos she confronts as she works out what it is to be whole person-oriented in her clinical work. Hospital specialist medicine is probably the arena of medical activity where biomedical reductionism is most obvious. Attracted to the MindBody approach and resolved to redress this reductionism, she is faced with her own developmental needs, questions of belonging, and MindBody skills limitations. It is enough to make one ill. Is the MindBody approach actually dangerous? Most aspiring MindBody healthcare clinicians know a good deal about these dilemmas, but few endure the pressures of confronting them in the major citadels of biomedicine. We are privileged to have this authentic and immediate account.

Leeanne Ford (Chapter eight) is a hospice nurse caring for the dying. She recounts the damaging effects of modern nursing practice upon a sensitive young woman who develops through mindfulness an admirable capacity to be present, and to act lovingly in that intimate space described by Mark Murphy; a space too often left closed or considered too difficult. Not without anxiety, but in a simple and practical way, Ford amplifies these spaces, recognizing and illustrating the moment-by-moment interpersonal nature of healthcare relationships, and the extraordinary meaningful and poignant transformational moments that arise when the nurse is fully present. The sheer simplicity of such moments beckons us all to deploy our humanity this way too. Indeed, MindBody work is a succession of such moments surrounded by all the usual tasks of orthodox healthcare.

Susan Lugton (Chapter nine) is a physiotherapist. For her, touch is not just a trained professional modality, but arises in and from an authentic desire to connect, relate, and finally heal. These dimensions of touch are stifled and deadened by the "training into the body as a predominantly biomedical, objective, and physical entity," with a consequent loss of the potential of touch as a healing modality. Lugton displays the honesty, candour, authenticity, and humanity of the MindBody clinician, and demonstrates the power and privilege of the body therapist who can be thoroughly present with both hands and ears. It is worth noting here that the majority of the contributors to this book are not psychotherapists or counsellors; they are other kinds of health professional who through their own transformations have discovered or reclaimed the power of listening and intimacy, of being more than usually present in the clinical encounter, and who now deploy these dimensions as a crucial element of their healing.

Sharon Wood (Chapter ten), a massage therapist, shows that her profession often disregard clients' personal stories, even though these are frequently evident and accessible. Body therapists may be restrained by unwillingness to engage in language interaction with patients, or lack the skills to do so, and emotional intimacy is often feared especially in the context of body contact. Wood's journey takes many years. She faces almost too many challenges, but in the end becomes, in my view, a fine clinician who can feel in the body what many people cannot; who can listen to stories in a way that few can; and who can create very safe intimate spaces for her clients to transform. In the end she listens with her ears and her hands comfortably integrated. Making the personal changes needed to become a MindBody clinician can be a long process, but it is clear that professional training, normative disciplinary paradigms, health system structures, and the real and perceived pressures from colleagues all operate to slow this process down. In other words the reductive paradigms stunt clinicians as human beings. Determined clinicians can break out of this, and systematic MindBody training and support greatly accelerates this change.

Julian Cloete (Chapter eleven) is a physiotherapist who has long been in pursuit of something else. By this he means that so often in practice the patient is presenting with something more than a painful elbow, or an injured knee. He is a curious man who takes pleasure in detective-work and loves the richness of whole person-oriented physiotherapy. He discovers that his natural bent towards this is greatly enhanced by adopting the phenomenological method. He absorbs insights and practices more commonly seen in psychotherapy practice and adapts them to his physiotherapy work, which becomes thereby much less reductive and more fulfilling. His contribution illustrates the reality that a clinician's original discipline and orthodoxy can be both maintained and greatly enhanced with a MindBody perspective.

Iona Winter (Chapter twelve) is a Maori psychotherapist, whose work is embedded in indigenous New Zealand culture. The idea of the connectedness of all things (very relevant to MindBody practice) is implicit in many aspects of Maori culture. In this view, the land, and spirit (wairua), and one's tupuna (forebears) are all represented in the therapy room, whether we care to notice or not. She draws attention to the disconnections that can occur when we move from traditional, intuitive and spiritual ways of sensing and knowing to more cognitive, intellectualized and disenchanted (Weber, 1964) frameworks. She wrestles with integration on multiple levels, and eventually achieves an inner coherence which at long last she can express in language, without losing the power of that which cannot be captured by language. In the MindBody approach we grapple with what we allow ourselves to see, hear, and recognize, and Winter's story will likely take some otherwise open readers out of their comfort zones. I suspect much of what she writes about has resonance with the visible and invisible stories behind the epidemic health problems of Maori in New Zealand.

Yvonne Evans (Chapter thirteen) is a narrative therapy-trained school guidance counsellor with a long, broad and senior experience in the education sector. It is sobering to see that the fragmentation due to modern Western reductionism pervades educational systems as much as it does healthcare. Again we see a strenuous journey away from impersonal systems-driven processes to determined person-centredness, demonstrated in the difficult context of working with often highly disadvantaged and traumatized young people in dysfunctional social systems. Is the body a rightful focus for non-health professionals working with young people? Negotiating professional boundaries, being able to explain lucidly what one is or is not doing, managing misunderstanding and holding steady in the face of this, and living with the isolation that can occur for whole person-oriented clinicians in a sea of people who function differently are all daily challenges for MindBody clinicians.

Marlies Dorrestein (Chapter fourteen) is a University lecturer in occupational therapy, and yet another clinician impelled to pursue person-centred care, partly because of previous serious personal illness. She is a teacher of student clinicians challenged by the question of what is most needed to foster person-centredness amongst her students and in her discipline. She draws on concepts of intimacy, lived body, and mindfulness to enable her process of change. Healing processes are mediated relationally, personal meanings and underpinning assumptions are excavated and examined, and life events are reconsidered. Healing is about the flow of healthy person-to-person influence, and the ripples affect patients, clients, trainees, students, colleagues; even friends and family.

Chris Cornelius (Chapter fifteen), a university academic in the social sciences, reflects on a lifetime of allergies and, in particular, severe eczema of the skin. There are two powerful strands in this chapter. In the first, he struggles with a chronic disease for decades, searching for biomedical help. The second strand is the story of a child who lost his mother; a story entirely invisible to his health providers over the decades of biomedical care. Yet it is this element that has been so potent in his life, and when this is addressed he begins to heal. Life experience, disease, and healing are all entwined, and the message is clear: in all chronic conditions, what are we not seeing and not responding to?

Peta Joyce (Chapter sixteen) provides a contrasting story, of a potentially lethal condition; breast cancer. Finding a clinician who can hold all the dimensions of her personhood while she tackles this grave challenge is impossible. Most clinicians deal with bits of the body and tender their favoured investigative and therapeutic modalities. She herself must hold the multidimensionality of her own personhood in the face of all the fragmentation of care and the splits between reductionist and whole person approaches. She does so, but it is a huge task. We are privileged to see what is possible for a person determined to adopt a whole person approach to a threatening illness. One is left pondering the fate of many others in similar situations but without her insights, skills, determination, and resourcefulness. Such people need clinicians with a MindBody approach who implicitly and explicitly embody a willingness to hold the patient multi-dimensionally.

Chris Hayes and Stephanie Oaks (Chapter seventeen) of the Hunter Integrative Pain Service, New South Wales, Australia, provide an admirable account of a large pain medicine team that honestly confronts the failure of the biomedical and biopsychosocial (Engel, 1977) models to provide pain treatments that meet the needs of patients, referring professionals, team clinicians, hospital management and funding authorities. From the beginning the leadership in this Pain Service aspire to a person-centred care and go on a rigorous, self-critical and determined ten year exploration. Eventually they adopt a story-based model of person-centred care, and their account of the in-team processes in moving to this are of great interest. For me, the outstanding features of this team transformation process are the visionary, persistent and wise leadership, the sense that the person-centred values of the story or MindBody approach with patients were also being enacted within the team and were part of the team transformation process; and finally the way the team as a group are able to hold the multidimensional complexity of good person-centred care. This is a land-mark example of MindBody transformation of a team in a mainstream medical discipline. We cannot dismiss the story or MindBody approach as merely the preserve of St Francis-like idealists. The MindBody approach is for all clinicians, because all clinicians are first and foremost persons, and when the approach is introduced in a wise, thoughtful, and unthreatening way, there is an attraction because the approach is intuitively right.

Finally, in the MindBody approach, the patient is first and foremost a person-in-relationship. Because difficult experiences in relationships can trigger illness and disease, the quality of the relationship with the healthcare professional plays a crucial role in healing. Good clinical care is a skillful blending of scientific knowledge and theory, and a deep respect for the clinical relationship and the power of generous empathy and professional kindness. Can clinicians learn to be expert in these ways? In this volume we see they can.

References

Antonovsky, A. (1979). *Health, stress and coping*. San Francisco: Jossey-Bass Publishers.

Antonovsky, A. (1996). The salutogenic model as a theory to guide health promotion. *Health promotion international 11(1)*: 11–18.

Antonovsky, A. (1987). *Unravelling the mystery of health—how people manage stress and stay well*. San Francisco: Jossey-Bass Publishers.

Broom, B. C. (1991). Somatisation: an endless epidemic. *Journal of Christian Health Care 4(1)*: 21–28.

Broom, B. C. (1997). *Somatic illness and the patient's other story. A practical integrative Mind/Body approach to disease for doctors and psychotherapists*. London: Free Association Books.

Broom, B. C. (2000). Medicine and story: a novel clinical panorama arising from a unitary mind/body approach to physical illness. *Advances in Mind/Body Medicine 16*: 161–207.

Broom, B. C. (2002). Somatic metaphor: a clinical phenomenon pointing to a new model of disease, personhood, and physical reality. *Advances in Mind/Body Medicine 18*: 16–29.

Broom, B. C. (2007). *Meaning-full disease: How personal experience and meanings initiate and maintain physical illness.* London: Karnac.

Broom, B. C. (2010). A reappraisal of the role of "mindbody" factors in chronic urticaria. *Postgrad Med J 86*: 365–370.

Broom, B. C., Booth, R. J. & Schubert, C. (2012). Symbolic illness and "mindbody" co-emergence. A challenge for psychoneuroimmunology. *Explore 8(1)*: 16–25.

Chiozza, L. A. (1998a). *Hidden affects in somatic disorders. Psychoanalytic perspectives on asthma, psoriasis, diabetes, cerebrovascular disease, and other disorders.* Madison, Connecticut: Psychosocial Press.

Chiozza, L. A. (1998b). *Why do we fall ill? The story hiding in the body.* Madison, Connecticut: Psychosocial Press.

Engel, G. L. (1977). The need for a new medical model: a challenge for biomedicine. *Science 196*: 129–136.

Groddeck, G. (1928). *The meaning of illness.* London: The Hogarth Press and the Institute of Psychoanalysis.

Hay, D. (1964). *The medieval centuries.* New York: Harper Torchbooks.

Heidegger, M. (1935). *The origin of the work of art. Poetry, language, thought.* New York: Harper and Row.

Heidegger, M. (1962). *Being and time.* New York: Harper and Row.

Levenson, E. A. (1974). Changing concepts of intimacy in psychoanalytic practice. *Contemporary Psychoanalysis 10*: 359–69.

Levinas, E. (1996). *Proper names.* Stanford: Stanford University Press.

Merleau-Ponty, M. (1969). *The visible and the invisible.* Place: Northwestern University Press.

Ricoeur, P. (1984). *Time and narrative.* London: The University of Chicago Press, Ltd.

Weber, M. (1964). *The sociology of religion.* Boston: Beacon Press.

CHAPTER TWO

The Kafka beetle goes off his food

Sharon Carey

'God!' he thought. 'What an exhausting job I've chosen. On the road day in and day out—much more stressful than working from home! And apart from the demands of doing business, the actual travelling is so bad: struggling to catch connecting trains, terrible meals at all hours of the day and night, a sea of ever-changing faces and never any chance of making friends. To hell with it all!'

—Franz Kafka, Metamorphosis, 1915

Disappointed and disheartened dietitian

Around school-leaving age I discovered human nutrition and dietetics, a profession offering a dynamic, practical and promising career in which I could pursue my two favourite subjects, human biology and home economics (food). After four years of university study I proudly emerged with an honours degree. For me, being a dietitian was symbolic of health and therefore an important achievement. Yet my career path did not match the youthful anticipation of an exciting vocation in nutrition. I soon felt stuck on a health service treadmill, and became disillusioned and, ironically, unwell. Where was my life heading? What was I doing here? Was I actually doing anything worthwhile? Gradually I changed from an energetic, enthusiastic and resourceful human being to a fatigued, dissatisfied and dispirited shell.

It would be inaccurate to describe my experience entirely negatively. I have enjoyed working in three countries, and in exciting city and friendly rural hospitals. I have been a community dietitian in the poorest and the most affluent suburbs in Auckland, and I have experienced the roller-coaster ride of private practice. I have consulted with hundreds of people presenting with a multitude of interesting health problems and nutrition-related queries. Eventually I found a niche as an immunology/allergy dietitian in a MindBody-oriented immunology department in a metropolitan hospital.

Yet, there remains the collateral story of disillusionment. I felt constricted by a dualistic, reductionist and materialist health culture which divides healthcare into body or mind disorders. I neither questioned nor dared step outside of what were considered to be my professional boundaries and dietetic scope of practice.

Professional boundaries are supposedly set to ensure safe practice and protect the clinician and patient. Without much insight, I believed I was working the correct way, especially as I deployed evidence-based methodologies. Yet despite significant literature skills I had never really learned to question the facts and the way we practised. I had chosen a career in which I could care for people, but there was no emphasis upon, or even recognition of what I now see as the relational space between the dietitian and patient.

With some shame I acknowledge that this narrow viewpoint was both ignorant and arrogant, especially as I was working obliviously with a reductionist, physicalist focus. I did not see the bigger picture. As Hungarian-British polymath Michael Polanyi (1967, p. 4) said, "We can know more than we can tell", that is, much of our learned behaviours are subconscious, and sometimes we are unable to translate our innermost knowing into words. Over time I began to develop an intangible desire for a different kind of practice. An unbearable internal conflict developed.

What I have learned

Postponing the story of my change process for the moment, I now see healthcare in a whole new light. I was enthralled to discover the denigrated placebo effect can be reinstated as a useful Meanings Response, and signifies a powerful set of processes highly relevant to healing (Moerman, 2002). Importantly, this phenomenon suggests that the clinician-patient relationship can, under various circumstances, offer more healing potential than a prescription. I have discovered that physical symptoms can be symbolic and meaningful (Broom, 1997, 2000, 2007; Chiozza, 1998a, 1998b; Groddeck, 1977; McDougall, 1989), and that the ability to discern such symbolism from both the body and language may play a key role in a clinician's healing skill base (Broom, Booth & Schubert, 2012; Broom, 2002; Griffith & Griffith, 1994). These insights suggest novel pathways to overcome chronic disorders unresponsive to the biomedical model.

I have also learned there is more than one truth. Our individual perceptions of the world are "learned phenomena" (Chopra, 2008, p. 22). For example, there is much more to food than just nutrient content. Food is obtained, prepared and eaten in socio-cultural contexts, and is therefore marinated in meaning. Thus the same food substances may affect different people in different ways, a phenomenon clearly germane to the controversial field of food hypersensitivity and intolerance. Narrow scientific cause-and-effect modelling may fail patients with these often perplexing food reactions unless these wider perspectives are entertained. I agree with Broom (2002, 2012) that a new, unitive MindBody model of disease that accommodates interacting truths and dimensions is required in healthcare.

I have come to value the uniqueness and individuality of each patient and their experience of illness and wellness. Reductionism corrals them into diagnostic groups, rendering invisible the richer truth of their individual reality and hindering healing. Taking a person-centred healthcare approach is of paramount importance and yet not commonplace.

The Cartesian (Descartes, 1641) splitting of the body (objectivity) and mind (subjectivity) makes it difficult to treat the whole person. Medicine treats the body like a car with parts that need to be fixed but does not focus on the car's journey. People enter the consulting room as whole persons with life-times of meaningful experiences rather than just as a body with broken parts. Blaise Pascal warned, "it's impossible to know the parts without studying the whole"(cited in Larson, 1999, p. 125).

I now understand that my experiences and story affect every patient I consult, and their stories shape my experiences, perceptions and clinical opinions. I cannot separate myself from my profession. I need the freedom to work authentically and humbly. This means letting down those apparently protective barriers that make us seem professional and powerful. Patients do not just seek our medical knowledge and opinions but our genuine respect and understanding.

I now recognise medicine to be symptom-focused rather than directed towards the deep-rooted origins of ill health. For example, by focussing on food triggers in the food-intolerant person, one is diverted from what is driving their hypersensitive state in the first place, commonly their underlying life story. Commonly-used food elimination diets may provide temporary sticking plasters to cover deep wounds of the past, eventually creating more problems than they resolve, including the ultimately anti-therapeutic potential to deter people from addressing the core of their experience.

To take a whole-person approach I needed to learn more about the mind. Although I studied psychology and sociology during my dietetics training, particularly to understand eating behaviours, the focus was upon using empirical science for a materialist understanding of nutrition and the human body. Philosophical topics such as meaning and spirituality were barely mentioned. Despite learning some good listening skills I did not learn how to listen deeply. I came to see clearly that reductionist scopes of practice make it difficult to ask certain questions, especially those of a personal nature. Clinicians typically avoid talking about their patients' feelings and emotions, let alone acknowledging that body, mind and spirit intertwine and flow as one entity, the MindBody.

A "Kafka beetle"

Dietetics, as I had learned it and saw it practised, did not work for me, and for years I was conflicted. I had embarked on a career symbolic of health and had morphed into a Kafka beetle (Kafka, 1915). I began my working life in a large, teaching hospital working long, demanding hours on hectic wards with inadequate resources. Within months, I seriously doubted my career choice. Whilst delighting in sharing my fresh nutrition knowledge and helping people recover from illness, I soon became irritated by the bureaucracy, tight budgets and inability to get the simplest of changes up-and-running, such as providing nourishing soup. I sensed the hopelessness of some patients and the frustration of relatives. My efforts felt inadequate, and I was soon exhausted. Had

I signed away my soul to the National Health Service? I had little time for being, thinking or caring. I was a cog in a large, crumbling wheel. Missing targets meant disappointing patients, which I found unbearable. There was under-resourcing and excessive expectation. I felt constricted, frustrated, and disheartened. I was hopeful that the health service might be different in New Zealand, but found there were similar expectations and politics, fewer resources (though fewer patients).

In Kafka's story, the salesman wakes one day as an unrecognisable, grotesque beetle, trapped in a hopeless situation, and abandoned by his colleagues and family. I was too busy to notice that my health was slowly deteriorating. I reached my lowest point on medical wards in an Auckland hospital. I became trapped within an anxiety-driven cycle of thinking. I could not work out whether my new supposed "depression problem" caused me to dislike my job or if my job made me feel so lost and miserable. For many months, I cried to *myself* as I journeyed to work. I did not have the capacity to talk to anyone about how I felt. My unimpressed colleagues eventually noticed I was becoming withdrawn and regarded me as "over-sensitive". I felt misunderstood, isolated, hopeless and dreadful. I was not me anymore.

Was my work in healthcare making me ill? Despite little recognition, I often worked late, struggling to keep up with the day-to-day patient care. I resented spending the majority of my time and skills trying to tempt sick people with unappetising hospital food and even more unappetising nutrition supplement drinks. Early nutrition intervention in people at risk of malnutrition reduces the risk of failure to thrive, medical complications, and the length of hospital stay; at least in the short-term (Barker, Gout & Crowe, 2011; Milne, Potter, Vivanti & Avenell, 2006). Thriving is more than adequate kilojoules and protein. I sensed that many of my patients needed my acknowledgement and tender loving care. There was no time for talking as the referrals for poor appetite and weight loss flooded in.

I reflect now on Viktor Frankl's discussion of what it took to survive the horrors of Auschwitz (Frankl, 2006). Despite the widespread suffering of severe malnutrition in dire and terrifying circumstances, some people were fuelled by something else which enabled them to persevere. Frankl thought that self-respecting people who allowed their suffering to be meaningful possessed an inner strength. Those with an optimistic outlook, or who held on to love, found the strength to survive despite all odds.

Iwaniac (2004) studied failure to thrive in children. He noticed that non-organic factors such as neglect impacted on health and wellbeing. People need to feel loving-kindness and human touch. Harlow (1958) completed ground-breaking work that showed infant rhesus monkeys bonded with soft, terrycloth surrogate mothers who did not offer food, rather than wire surrogate mothers with milk. From a broader nutrition perspective, the context in which nutritious food is eaten in, and the influence of this, may have a significant impact on health and one's ability to thrive. "What makes for a straighter spine, vitamin D or self-esteem?" (Chopra, 2008, p. 141).

In hindsight, I found working on surgical wards more fulfilling than working on medical wards because people with sometimes straight-forward, organic problems could be successfully treated. In these contexts, nutrition intervention was clearly beneficial. The end-result was visible and often rewarding. However the picture was different upon medical wards. Although I knew my dietary advice was somewhat helpful for chronically-ill patients, I sensed their despair. Like many of them I felt burdened, fatigued and unhappy. Despite being young and apparently fit, I too was failing to thrive.

I know that, in part, this downward spiral in my health resulted from working in an inauthentic way. I was in a constant state of doing, not being, dredging through vast to-do lists. I rarely experienced the present moment, the Now (Tolle, 1999). I merely existed, and did not feel alive anymore. In my immaturity, I sacrificed my self-care while caring for others. I had not learned how to set appropriate boundaries or how to assert myself. I was eager to perform and unable to easily say "no".

Since my MindBody training I have come to realize that some of my ill-health experience resulted from transference and counter-transference. I am referring particularly to the fascinating phenomenon of sensing the patient's experiences and affect in one's own body (Stone, 2006). I naturally attune to people. I am intuitive and sensitive, and, when I struggled in my work, I assumed I lacked the broad shoulders required for coping with the demands of hospital-based care. It is now clear that as I empathically listened to my patients I took on their experiences both emotionally and physically. I did not know how to use this data to help me understand my patients' bodied experiences. I took their illnesses home with me and in me. I now realize that personal psychotherapy and professional supervision can be crucial in managing one's own health whilst working to improve that of others. Use of these resources is routine and even mandatory for psychotherapists and social workers. Yet where supervision is accessed by body-focussed practitioners, it seems to be focussed upon professional "skills" rather than upon problematic feelings and the more subtle and complex phenomena that arise in the inter-subjective space between clinician and patient.

What did I do with my unhappiness? I changed my job several times in the hope of feeling better. I particularly enjoyed working as a community dietitian. Away from acute care medicine I had more chance to be myself. I took opportunities to listen compassionately, and work with patients as whole persons rather than as bodies with parts. Community care tends to be more holistic than in acute hospital care, though the term holistic is often construed as meaning unscientific and unprofessional. On the contrary, holism means treating the whole person, and all dimensions of the person as one. Once there were just doctors, nurses and physiotherapists but now we have a different health professional for every aspect of human personhood. As our scopes of practice have reduced so our opportunities for working holistically have diminished.

Eventually, I decided to escape the confines of publicly-funded healthcare and work in private practice. At last I was free to think for myself and allow more time per consultation. This was an exciting yet exhausting period. The hours were long and the money hard-earned. But it allowed more creativity and fulfilment.

During this time I learned how to overcome my anxiety state through the use of cognitive behavioural therapy techniques, yet I did not address the meaning of my poor health. I did not listen to the message it was bringing. I learned how to control the anxiety and, in the process, unconsciously swapped the anxiety for another chronic state; pain.

From unconsciousness to consciousness

The pain crept up on me. One day it occurred to me that I had been suffering ongoing aches and pains. A friend complained of his sore knee and I thought, "What is he moaning about? For a long time I have had had stiff, aching joints, all over my body yet I do not complain about them". Sometimes I could hardly move my back, as though the muscles had been glued together. I felt like a scarecrow with a steel rod down my spine and another across my shoulder blades, rendering me inflexible. I felt "crushed" and "stuck". These metaphors bear great significance now although I did not interpret them at the time.

I had previously seldom visited doctors, but that all changed. I got to experience being a disempowered and discontented patient. I can now appreciate why some people appear so disgruntled with health services. I had always respected and trusted health professionals but my patience soon wore thin. I felt misunderstood, and generally disrespected as a human being presenting with a lived experience and a failing body. The more my symptoms were treated dualistically, the sicker I became. The diagnostic dots would not join up, leaving me confused and searching for answers. Why could (or would) no-one help me?

The pain in my joints and muscles became more widespread and severe. I assumed they had resulted from sporting activities. Physiotherapy did not relieve them. A massage therapist did suggest the muscle tension might be related to stress. I developed recurrent chest infections and asthma following common colds. I assumed this was secondary to exposure to new germs in a new country.

I ended up with a ridiculous collection of inhalers. I remember feeling angered by the asthma specialist nurse who said that I would need to be on a strict daily inhaler regimen for the rest of my life. This did not make sense because I only suffered "asthma" for a few months in the winter following colds, and antibiotics seemed to do a much better job of resolving it. I sensed some form of misdiagnosis.

I was labelled as asthmatic, and non-compliant at that. I considered myself to be a reasonably well person who was merely vulnerable to asthmatic episodes in the winter. This demonstrates how labelling someone with an illness, because their symptoms loosely follow a pattern, can cast them into a sick box. A person-centred view would have focussed on my experience, not my compliance with a diagnosis. Labels can be reductionist and disempowering, and may paradoxically encourage ill health.

I sensed my doctor did not want to be bothered by my invisible health problem. I wanted reassurance that I was not going mad, yet I felt like a thirty-something neurotic female in his office, despite knowing I was genuinely suffering. My (male) friend, who had the same GP, was booked without fuss for surgery, yet I was not referred to any specialist. The sense of isolation caused my mood to drop. I became self-blaming for my misery pains. The more I tried to fathom what was happening, the more it fed the anxiety, and the worse I got. I was trapped and the pain, stiffness and exhaustion amplified.

During the worst of my experience, I felt utterly fatigued. My muscles felt weak and useless, and the effort of moving was like wading through treacle. My head felt fog-like and regular tension headaches and migraines incapacitated me. Occasionally I would jump due to a sensation of hot prickles on my skin. It felt as though my nervous system was buzzing with electricity. I was hypersensitive to touch, light, noise, odours and eventually certain strongly flavoured foods. I felt wound up and my tolerance threshold was low. My sleep did not refresh me. As the chronic fatigue and stiffness set in, I felt I was rapidly aging, and that part of me had died.

I was eventually diagnosed with fibromyalgia. My doctor informed me that I would suffer chronic, worsening pain for the rest of my life and that there was not really anything that could be done for me. He suggested I would need to be about as fit as someone who could complete the Ironman endurance event to feel better, yet I could barely get out of bed. His colleague suggested some bizarre alternative treatment that heated or cooled my blood.

I did not feel I was being taken seriously. A simple acknowledgement of my suffering would have been far more helpful, but my doctor reminded me that his office was "not the place for talking about feelings". I felt infuriated, powerless, despondent, depressed and deeply ashamed to have failed somehow. I hid my suffering, particularly from my medical colleagues.

In an attempt to cheer myself up and overcome my misery pains I resumed some old hobbies. I recommenced trumpet lessons but lacked the puff to play. I returned to dance classes but just one practice session could land me in bed for hours, seized up like a rusted robot. I considered yoga for flexibility and relaxation but could not find the time or energy. The more I attempted to do, the worse I got.

Eventually, a unitary approach which acknowledged experiences and personal meanings helped me to overcome a medical condition that apparently has no cure. I started to recognize that my body was symbolically expressing what I was unable to language. My symptoms symbolized my feeling of being stuck. I felt crushed from the pressure I was under both professionally and personally. Although I needed to slow down and live more authentically I was too busy doing to stop and listen. My body made me stop. I eventually had to acknowledge its messages.

I realized I needed more psychological therapy to understand the connection. Yet I was seeking help at the other end of a dualistic health-care spectrum. The process of finding a therapist I could gel with was expensive and arduous. Many of the therapists I met focussed on the mind and emotions, and did not talk about the bodied, physical experience of fibromyalgia. I gained precious insight about myself and felt less depressed, although I still suffered with pain and stiffness. Then I crossed paths with two MindBody-oriented practitioners and my life encountered a miraculous turn-around.

MindBody therapy healed my fibromyalgia in two consultations

These MindBody practitioners were comfortable with talking about the mind and body. Their humanistic approach was centred round my experience. I was given the opportunity to explore the personal meanings to my symptoms as I was gently mobilized on a self-healing journey.

The first health professional is a physician/psychotherapist. He is my colleague, not my therapist. I felt "stuck" in supporting some food-hypersensitive patients who did not respond to dietary measures. My colleague educated me about symbolism, personal meanings and somatisation. This MindBody enlightenment enabled me to notice my symptoms as symbolic and meaningful.

Around this time I also found a suitable therapist. He is a psychologist/mindfulness expert. Together we explored the personal meanings my symptoms represented, and discussed the difficulties I was experiencing in life. Of course some of these were of a personal nature; life experiences that dated back to childhood that needed to be processed; but a lot had to do with my encounters working in a sick healthcare system. I finally understood why I needed to slow down.

At last I felt respectfully treated. I no longer felt disempowered because I was treated as an equal in a non-judgmental way. This connection made me feel less isolated, which caused my mood to lift immediately. The all-over body stiffness and pain effortlessly disintegrated. My energy level noticeably increased and within six months I had run a half-marathon. I rarely suffer asthma symptoms and seldom use inhalers. I felt alive again.

I still experience the odd twinge via a stiff neck or headache but now read the signals and know when to stop. I overcame an incurable, chronic condition and feel more healthy and optimistic than ever before.

I still have occasional maintenance therapy with my psychologist, whom I trust and respect, and this gives me the opportunity for self-reflection and personal development. I am very fortunate to receive professional supervision with my psychotherapist colleague at work, discussing the management of difficult cases and ways that I can develop my skills and patient service. I can also, importantly, attend to self-care. I am very proud of the recovery I made and the stronger person and better health professional I have become. I have evolved into a MindBody oriented dietitian and my clinical practice has transformed.

Finally, though at first I was hesitant to disclose my use of psychotherapy, for fear of being judged, I am now open about it. Unfortunately, even in healthcare, there is much stigma unduly attached to using psychological therapies. It is often misunderstood, as if you have a weakness. However, using psychotherapy demonstrates a strength showing motivation to understand more about your true, undisguised self.

Integrating MindBody practice in hospital outpatient clinical care

As I widened my focus to see story-and-meaning in my work with patients, I noticed a lot of symbolism in my immunology-dietary outpatient clinics. My aim shifted from deploying specialized diets towards bringing about new insight and awareness in my patients. I meet many frustrated food-hypersensitive patients with conditions such as Irritable Bowel Syndrome (IBS), chronic urticaria (hives) and occasionally terrifying anaphylaxis-like adverse reactions. By taking a whole-person rather than diet-focussed approach I have come closer to uncovering the root causes that drive these hypersensitivity states. Some patients, who make these new connections between their life story and symptoms, rapidly overcome long histories of food intolerance as they change their focus.

The underlying mechanisms of food hypersensitivity are often complex and may include allergic reactions, cumulative unexplained intolerances, and learned or conditioned responses. Most of what is driving the hypersensitive state appears to be at a subconscious level, although problem food substances (natural or added) are often blamed. Food intolerance is a symptom, not a root cause of ill health. There is no doubt certain food substances can cause adverse reactions for some people but this does not acknowledge why. Why would an everyday food such as bread, milk or fruit cause such illness in one person but not in the next? Why has that person become intolerant to something basic and necessary? One way of looking at this is that if there is something that has the potential to make you stop and take account of your life it is the inability to eat.

The scientific evidence is lacking for the use of food elimination diets in many of the food intolerance and other syndromes to which they are applied, and I have found that food-focussed sufferers frequently get stuck on an elimination pathway, which ultimately results in bland, unbalanced and expensive diets and poor long-term benefits to health. The more experience I gained in this fascinating field the more I was convinced that food elimination diets were not the long-term answer to resolving food hypersensitivity. This is the general viewpoint of the immunology department I work within.

My particular interest is directed towards the common condition of IBS. It costs countries billions of dollars in expensive medical tests, sub-optimal treatments and absenteeism from work (Inadomi, Fennerty & Bjorkman, 2003). It appears that IBS is driven by central autonomic dys-regulation and visceral hypersensitivity, in other words it is a sensitivity state (Tillisch, Mayer & Labus, 2011; Elsenbruch, et al., 2010; Agrarwal et al., 2008; Crowell, 2004; Mertz, 2003; Gupta, Sheffield & Verne, 2002; Houghton, Cooper, Jackson & Whorwell, 2002; Drossman, 1996). Little is known about how to down-regulate this hypersensitivity. Perhaps the irritable bowel represents the body's urgent demand for attention, like an "intuitive barometer"? I hypothesize that a unitary treatment approach that addresses life experiences and personal meanings could finally be the answer to long-term healing.

It is well documented that emotional states such as anger, anxiety, tension, excitement, sadness, hopelessness and relaxation affect the sensitivity of the gut (Beesley, Rhodes & Salmon, 2010; Elsenbruch, et al., 2010; Muscatello, et al., 2010; Houghton, Calvert & Jackson, 2002; Kiecolt-Glaser & Newton, 2001; Blomhoff et al., 2000; Houghton et al., 1995; Whorwell & Houghton, 1992). Emotionally-laden life events such as past or current physical, emotional and/or sexual abuse can increase the risk of IBS, although a biomedical approach may not see this (Beesley et al 2010; Wilson, 2010; Rey & Talley, 2009; Moore, 2009; Pae, Masand, Ajwani, Lee & Patkar, 2007; Dreher 2003; Creed, Craig & Farmer, 1988). Conflict increases the risk of IBS whereas feeling supported, particularly by one's spouse, reduces it (Gerson et al., 2006; Kiecolt-Glaser & Newton, 2001; Creed et al., 1988).

An exclusion diet, such as the modish low FODMAP diet (Shepherd & Gibson, 2006; Gibson & Shepherd, 2010), may provide temporary relief of symptoms but will not resolve visceral hypersensitivity. On the other hand, a key tool for healing is an empathic, genuine, person-centred therapeutic relationship (Frenkel, 2008; Moore, 2008; Walach & Jonas, 2004; Moerman, 2002; Broom, 2002).

I enhance my dietetic skills by applying integrative, interpersonal therapeutic techniques. I have expanded my listening skills and ability to build rapport. I make use of the meanings response (Moerman, 2002) and transference/countertransference (Stone, 2006). I carefully consider language and metaphor. I try to accompany a patient on their self-healing journey, rather than dutifully fixing them with a diet. I still comply with the biomedical framework, yet with a MindBody-orientation. This all takes time and patience.

I now help people recognize they may need to peel back many layers to reach the core of their illness. I am not trained to offer psychotherapy, although I find myself developing these skills. It is regrettable that our health service does not fund enough therapists, let alone those with a MindBody perspective. I help people to understand their illness as meaning-full, and explore their story with them. I act as a catalyst to help my patients enhance self-awareness and ultimately experience a shift in consciousness. This empowers self-healing and helps people recognize where ongoing therapy may be beneficial, overcoming the stigma attached to receiving it.

Here are two examples of how I may work with patients suffering food hypersensitivity.

> A twenty-eight-year old woman, who I shall call Amanda, with a ten year history of IBS was referred to me after extensive, expensive and invasive medical investigations ruled out organic disease. She was convinced that something sinister was happening in her bowel and furious that "the doctors could find nothing wrong and think it's all in my head" (a statement I often hear). Amanda suffered problematic fluctuating bowel motions in combination with excruciating abdominal pain, lingering back ache and lethargy. She had low self-esteem and a sad lament.
>
> I first took a standard dietary approach and supported Amanda in following the food chemical exclusion diet that the doctor requested. Although Amanda complied with the bland diet for more than a month her symptoms persisted. Upon review she was convinced she must have coeliac disease, despite negative coeliac

serology. I next provided a tailored meal plan and low FODMAP diet (Gibson & Shepherd, 2010, 2006) which is reduced in fermentable carbohydrate-containing foods such as wheat, although not as strict as a gluten-free diet.

It was important for Amanda to trust me so I carefully worked on building rapport at each meeting. She was already experiencing a theme of feeling like she was not taken seriously by the doctors and by work colleagues who were bullying her. This was going to be a slow process and patience was paramount.

After another month I reviewed Amanda's progress. She found some relief on the low FODMAP diet, which is a low wind-making diet. I could have discharged Amanda on a low FODMAP, modified fibre diet but she was on a dangerous pathway of dietary restriction. Amanda was underweight, over-exercising and "scared of getting fat".

Interestingly, Amanda's food focus had shifted. She no longer believed she had coeliac disease. Rapport had been built and a great opportunity for MindBody intervention had arisen. I carefully listened and curiously enquired. I asked questions outside the nutrition box to find out more about her story. Amanda had suffered stomach migraine in early childhood. Her IBS symptoms worsened when she left home; that important time when one first tests the life-coping skills one learns in childhood. It emerged that Amanda had suffered childhood abuse—where the theme of not being taken seriously appeared to have its roots.

Amanda had had counselling in the past and noticed her IBS symptoms had improved when taking antidepressants. This is not surprising because selective serotonin reuptake inhibitors work on the serotonin in the gastrointestinal tract as well as the brain. Amanda finally understood that her gut was acting like an intuitive barometer. She accepted that she had embodied her experience and that suppressed emotions were affecting her gastrointestinal health. Her miserable working situation had triggered those buried feelings.

Several months later, during my final review, Amanda reported feeling much better. She had just started psychotherapy and had left her office job in favour of a horticultural career. She appeared happier and more energetic than previously, and had managed to significantly relax her dietary restrictions. Food was no longer her focus; she was free of her demons and in control of her health.

Barbara presented with a complex history of chronic urticaria and angioedema, eczema, IBS and multiple food and drug intolerances. I sensed her anxiety, which she was trying to hide. Rather than focusing on food elimination diets I listened empathically to Barbara's story. She opened up about her difficult childhood and currently difficult relationship. I did not attempt psychotherapy as I do not have such skills. However I am able to comfortably listen without passing judgement, and acknowledged with her the fear, confusion and deep sadness that I sensed. Barbara lived in a family, society and culture where it was impossible for her to speak up, and so she buried her experiences within. Despite multiple food intolerances, a strict elimination diet was not going to repair the wounds of her past. After our first consultation she gave me this feed-back:

"Thank you so much. I just want you to know that I think God blessed me to meet you. You told me what I knew in my heart but there was no one around to understand that, and I really thank you for stepping outside of the norm, not just for me but others like me. You have no idea how much it's meant."

I speak enthusiastically about my MindBody discoveries to colleagues, family and friends. Some people seem to be relieved to hear my story and are eager to find out more. Yet others look bemused or uncertain. When I mention the word holistic some of my colleagues look at me with a dismissive expression.

Some colleagues have responded that "dietitians are not qualified to provide psychotherapy". They are correct. I have simply broadened my listening skills and taken a unitary approachs. Some of my colleagues in the health profession believed they were already providing such a service. I have heard responses such as, "yeah, yeah, I'm a good listener" or "I already give counselling". In such circumstances I felt annoyed that I had not actually been listened to at all by these people. They had purely made assumptions about the way I practice. I was not heard and I am sure their patients would have felt the same way. So often people with specialist knowledge like to offer expert opinions which are based upon their personal perceptions and the literature they have read. This is talking, not listening. It represents their own truths, not those of the patient.

Sometimes my efforts to help someone understand their core experiences are derailed by colleagues or patient family members who have a biomedical focus. This can be an incredibly frustrating step backwards, especially if yet another form of elimination diet is suggested. Dualistic socio-cultural influences can hinder the therapeutic process.

I have faced defensive colleagues and some soon realise, with some shame, they have their own self-care to attend to. Some have dedicated so much time and energy on their healthcare improvement-projects that the suggestion of a new way of doing things may be too overwhelming to bear. I was apprehensive at first when I learned about the meanings response and how this knowledge would change my worldview. Encouraging a biomedically-focussed co-worker to change their beliefs and see through a MindBody lens can be exhausting; like asking somebody to swap religions. I take refuge in a MindBody-focussed department.

When I looked at the world through this new panoramic lens I awakened to a new understanding of chronic ill health. My own personal MindBody experiences have been highly conditioned by my working in a healthcare system I was feeling crushed by. I was an ordinary person trying to survive an accelerating world of over-expectation. I know first hand what it is like to be a patient who feels let down and misunderstood by those I sought expert advice from; those same health professionals I have worked alongside for so long. I have experienced how the biomedical model can label one as chronically ill, perversely encouraging one to remain in a sick role, rather than promote the belief and ability to heal.

MindBody therapy has transformed my health, my healthcare practice and therefore the people around me. I have a helpful, non-judgmental attitude to working with people with functional and chronic health problems because I take morbidity as seriously as mortality. I am now more attracted to medicine than surgery, as I no longer feel the same need to fix people but I am learning to patiently accompany them on their self-healing journey.

In my role as a MindBody-oriented specialist immunology dietitian I am fortunate to find meaning in helping other people find meaning. I love my optimistic job. I joined the health service so I could help people feel better, and that is what I often do. I have witnessed many moments of enlightenment and relief as some people, who adopt a meanings-perspective, realize they may be able to overcome nagging or debilitating health problems. Nonetheless, a whole-person approach in a dualistic health culture does not come without challenges. I certainly resonate with Mahatma Ghandi's exhortation; to be the change I wish to see in the world.

References

Agrarwal, A., Houghton, L., Lea, R., Morris, J., Reilly, B. & Whorwell, P. (2008). Bloating and distension in irritable bowel syndrome: The Role of Visceral Sensation. *Gastroenterology 134*: 1882–9.

Barker, L., Gout, B. & Crowe, T. (2011). Hospital malnutrition: prevalence, identification and impact on patients and the healthcare system. *International Journal of Environmental Research and Public Health 8*: 514–27.

Beesley, H., Rhodes, J. & Salmon, P. (2010). Anger and childhood sexual abuse are independently associated with irritable bowel syndrome. *British Journal of Psychology 15*: 389–99.

Blomhoff, S., Spetalen, S., Jacobsen, M., Vatn, M. & Malt, U. (2000). Intestinal reactivity to words with emotional content and brain information processing in irritable bowel syndrome. *Digestive Diseases and Sciences 45(6)*: 1160–5.

Broom, B. (1997). *Somatic illness and the patient's other story: a practical integrative approach to disease for doctors and psychotherapists*. New York/London: Free Association Books.

Broom, B. (2000). Medicine and story: a novel clinical panorama arising from a unitary Mind/Body approach to physical illness. *Advances in Mind-Body Medicine 16*: 161–207.

Broom, B. (2002). Somatic metaphor: a clinical phenomenon pointing to a new model of disease, personhood, and physical reality. *Advances in Mind-Body Medicine 18*: 16–29.

Broom, B. (2007). *Meaning-Full disease: how personal experience and meanings initiate and maintain physical illness*. London: Karnac.

Broom, B., Booth, R. & Schubert, C. (2012). Symbolic diseases and "Mindbody" co-emergence. A challenge for psychoneuroimmunology. *Explore 8(1)*: 16–25

Chiozza, L. (1998 a). *Hidden affects in somatic disorders. Psychoanalytic perspectives on asthma, psoriasis, diabetes, cerebrovascular disease, and other disorders*. Madison, Connecticut: Psychosocial Press.

Chiozza, L. (1998 b). *Why do we fall ill? The story hiding in the body*. Madison, Connecticut: Psychosocial Press.

Chopra, D. (2008). *Ageless body, timeless mind.* London: Rider

Creed, F., Craig, T. & Farmer, R. (1988). Functional abdominal pain, psychiatric illness and life events. *Gut 29(2)*: 235–42.

Crowell, M. (2004). Role of serotonin in the pathophysiology of the irritable bowel syndrome—review. *British Journal of Pharmacology 141(8)*: 1285–9.

Dreher, H (2003). *Mind-Body unity: A new vision for Mind-Body science and medicine.* Baltimore: John Hopkins University Press.

Descartes, R. (1641). Meditations on First Philosophy, in *The philosophical writings of René Descartes*, trans. by Cottingham J, Stoothoff R and Murdoch D, Cambridge: Cambridge University Press, 1984, vol 2, pp. 1–62.

Drossman, D. (1996). Gastrointestinal illness and the biopsychosocial model. *Journal of Clinical Gastroenterology Jun 22(4)*: 252–4.

Elsenbruch, S., Rosenberger, C., Enck, P., Forsting, M., Schedlowski, M. & Gizewski, E. (2010). Affective disturbances modulate the neural processing of visceral pain stimuli in irritable bowel syndrome: An fMRI study. *Gut 59*: 489–95.

Frankl, V. E. (2006). *Man's search for meaning.* Boston, USA: Beacon Press.

Frenkel, O. (2008). A Phenomenology of the "Placebo Effect": taking meaning from the mind to the body. *Journal of Medicine and Philosophy 33*: 58–79.

Gerson, M., Gerson, C., Awad, R., Dancey, C., Poitras, P., Porcelli, P. & Sperber, A. (2006). An international study of irritable bowel syndrome: family relationships and Mind-body attributions. *Social Science & Medicine 62*: 2838–47.

Gibson, P., Shepherd, S. (2010). Evidence-based dietary management of functional gastrointestinal symptoms: The FODMAP approach. *Journal of Gastroenterology and Hepatology 25*: 252–8.

Griffith, J. & Griffith, M. (1994). *The body speaks. Therapeutic dialogue for Mind-Body problems.* New York: Basic Books.

Groddeck, G. (1977). *The meaning of illness, selected psychoanalytic writings* (English Translation). International Psychoanalytical Library No 105, MMR Khan ed. London, The Hogarth Press, and The Institute of Psychoanalysis.

Gupta, V., Sheffield, D. & Verne, G. (2002). Evidence for autonomic dysregulation in the irritable bowel syndrome. *Digestive Diseases and Sciences 47(8)*: 1716–22.

Harlow, H. (1958). The nature of love. *American Psychologist 13*: 573–685.

Houghton, L., Calvert, E. & Jackson, N. (2002). Visceral sensation and emotion: A study using hypnosis. *Gut 51*: 701–4.

Houghton, L., Cooper, P., Jackson, N. & Whorwell, P. (1995). Visceral sensation and emotion: A study using hypnosis. *Gastroenterology 108 (4, Suppl 2)*: p. A618.

Inadomi, J., Fennerty, M. & Bjorkman, D. (2003). Systematic review: The economic impact of irritable bowel syndrome. *Alimentary Pharmacology and Therapeutics Oct 18(7)*: 671–82.

Iwaniec, D. (2004). *Children who fail to thrive: A practice guide*. Chichester, England: John Wiley & Sons.

Kafka, F. (1915). *The Metamorphosis*. Translated by W. Aaltonen. London: Arcturus Publishing Ltd., 2009.

Kiecolt-Glaser, J. & Newton, T. (2001). Marriage and health: his and hers. *Psychological Bulletin 127(4)*: 472–503.

Larson, J. (1999). The conceptualization of health. *Medical Care Research and Review 56(123)*: 123–36.

McDougall, J. (1989). *Theatres of the body. A psychoanalytic approach to psychosomatic illness*. London: Free Association Books.

Mertz, H. (2003). Review article: visceral hypersensitivity. *Alimentary Pharmacology & Therapeutics 17*: 623–33.

Milne, A., Potter, J., Vivanti, A. & Avenell, A. (2006). Protein and energy supplementation in elderly people at risk from malnutrition: a review. *The Cochrane Database of Systematic Reviews* (Issue 2).

Moerman, D. (2002). *Meaning, medicine and the "Placebo Effect"*. Cambridge: Cambridge University Press.

Moore, J. (2008). Uncovering the link between irritable bowel syndrome and abuse. *Kai Tiaki Nursing New Zealand 14(70)*: 22–3.

Muscatello, M., Bruno, A., Pandolfo, G., Mico, U., Stilo, S., Scaffidi, M., Consolo, P., Tortora, A., Pallio, S., Giacobbe, G., Familiari, L. & Zoccali, R. (2010). Depression, anxiety and anger in subtypes of irritable bowel syndrome. *Journal of Clinical Psychology in Medical Settings 17*: 61–70.

Pae, C., Masand, P., Ajwani, N., Lee, C. & Patkar, A. (2007). Irritable bowel syndrome in psychiatric perspectives: A comprehensive review. *International Journal of Clinical Practice 61(10)*: 1708–18.

Polanyi, M. (1966). *The Tacitdimension*. New York: Doubleday & Company, Inc.

Rey, E. & Talley, N. (2009). Irritable bowel syndrome: novel views on the epidemiology and potential risk factors. *Digestive and Liver Disease 41*: 772–80.

Shepherd, S. & Gibson, M. (2006). Fructose malabsorption and symptoms of irritable bowel syndrome: guidelines for effective dietary management. *Journal of the American Dietetic Association 106(10)*: 1631–9.

Stone, M. (2006). The analyst's body as tuning fork: embodied resonance in countertransference. *Journal of Analytical Psychology 51(1)*: 109–24.

Tillisch, K., Mayer, E. & Labus, J. (2011). Quantitative meta-analysis identifies brain Regions Activated During Rectal Distension in Irritable Bowel Syndrome. *Gastroenterology 140(1)*: 91–100.

Tolle, E. (1999). *The Power of Now: A guide to spiritual enlightenment.* Novato, CA. New World Library.

Walach, H. & Jonas, W. (2004). Placebo research: the evidence base for harnessing self-healing capacities. *The Journal of Alternative and Complementary Medicine 10*: S-103–12.

Whorwell, P. & Houghton, L. (1992). Physiological effects of emotion: assessment via hypnosis. *Lancet 340 (8811)*: 69–72.

Wilson, D. (2010). Health consequences of childhood sexual abuse. *Perspectives in Psychiatric Care 46(1)*: 56–64.

CHAPTER THREE

An intimate field

Mark Murphy

In this chapter I outline my integrative approach as a gestalt therapist, focussing on the philosophy and practice of dialogue. I argue that acknowledging our wholeness as persons with each other—mind, spirit, and always body—involves working in a radically intimate field.

In praise of space

Around my body there is a deep space. This space is clear and still, but also alive and quite substantial. It extends in the world like a great round bowl from me to the other in the room. Today, the space I inhabit feels vast, like being at the bottom of a deep blue valley. When I open my eyes and measure the space, I am astonished the gap is so little: two metres, perhaps, between me and the other, and about forty centimetres inside, across my middle. A blackbird calls out from the garden beyond. Beneath her call the wind is rustling. The wind-chimes in the tree begin to ring. Each sound is a clear fresh presence, appearing for the first and the very last time.

Martin Heidegger, in his meditations on the question of being, wrote of a space he called the clearing:

> In the midst of beings as a whole an open place occurs. There is a clearing, a lighting …. Only this clearing grants and guarantees to us humans a passage to those beings that we ourselves are not, and access to the being that we ourselves are. (Heidegger, 1935, p. 53)

Heidegger does not specify "the clearing" as an actual experience, yet it seems so evocative and familiar at some level. For now, I wish to simply translate the clearing as space. I need space to clearly meet what is present and different, to experience the fullness of who I am in the moment, and to be with whatever emerges in an authentic, chosen way. I hear the blackbird calling from the garden beyond. Hearing this, I feel warmly contented and whole. The muscles in my neck and shoulders spontaneously relax. I smile. I am not the blackbird or the garden beyond, but the call is already inside me. I choose to stop and take this in.

The clearing is one path to wholeness. We reach the truth of what is, and what is emerging together, by turning to the experiential openness of the moment. As a trainee integrative psychotherapist, I was taught by Brian Broom to trust what the patient gives and says in their symptoms and words, rather than push for new information or insight. Our best ideas, theories, and MindBody techniques often get in the way of what is revealed in the space before us. Brian taught a holographic faith in the sufficiency of what is; that the whole is always already present in any one of its parts, particularly in the client's symptom and story (Broom, 1997, 2000, 2002, 2007). This holistic phenomenological view was extended in my gestalt training. Pay attention to the process of your being together with the client, with awareness on all levels of experience, including your kinaesthetic and present felt energetic sense. What you need to most know is here. Whenever I rush the process of being with a client, or find myself searching for a breakthrough MindBody technique, I have left the clearing for the woods. The space between the client and me becomes cluttered, and I miss the richness of what is actually happening.

Where being comes into presence

The clearing provides a passage to the "being" that "we ourselves are"; and at the same time, to the "beings" that "we ourselves are not". The same "passage" through which we discover ourselves, we discover who (and "where") we are not as well. This insight is pivotal to how I have come to understand what it means to be present, to be whole or becoming whole as a person, and to work in a way that deeply acknowledges both our connectedness and separateness on many levels of our being, mind, body, and spirit.

Let me state that pivotal insight again. In the midst of beings as whole, there is space; a clearing in the trees, if you like, which provides a passage-way to the being that we are and to the beings that we are not. I love these words of Heidegger's. I believe they can offer a unique perspective on working holistically. Then I remember Heidegger's involvement with the National Socialist Party for a brief time during World War II, and I feel a deep discomfort as well. The basic argument I want to reinforce here is this; we are never mind, body, or spirit in an isolated way. Our wholeness emerges in relationship, in an intimate field.[1] Self and other emerge in the same moment, and in a powerfully physical way. This is miraculous and also dangerous. The fact that we emerge together is no guarantee as to how we will then respond.

In a way, the controversy over Heidegger's involvement with the National Socialist Party has nothing substantial to do with MindBody healthcare. Yet, in another way, it gestures to something else that is present in our field; our capacity for distrust and fear, and thereby a want to control and objectify what is unknown, different or other. Most clients I work with do not trust their bodies in a basic sense. Even speaking this way, as if "I" and "my body" are separate, illustrates the scar, or what Morris Berman (following Balint) calls the basic fault (Berman, 1989). In the West, at least, there is a deep, historical distrust that matter and body (and animals and the earth) are animated with vital life, with spirit or self, or are life-being and life-disclosing in an essential way. Worse, that the body (or the earth etc.) becomes a transference object for all that I cannot control or master, or worse again, for that which I can or I think I can control and master. The body is then treated as an achievement of the self, a vehicle for the self, or an unfortunate dragging chain and ball around the mind, self, and spirit. In the Jewish philosopher Martin Buber's elemental words, the body is not included as an essential part of I and You, but treated as an It: an object for our "goal-directed verbs" (Buber, 1923, p. 54).[2]

I think all of us live with the danger of turning our clients into objects for our goal-directed verbs. I am regularly drawn into wanting to do something, to achieve some therapeutic purpose or goal; alleviate depression, settle anxiety, cool off an irritable bowel and so on.

This, according to Buber, is the world of I and It; purposeful, useful, utilitarian, and inevitably part of how we function every day in the world. We get things done, I do this or that, I read a client through a framework of ideas, I aim for a certain therapeutic outcome with this or that person. The problem is not that we do this, but that we have come to place such a primary, and sometimes exclusive, value on this way of being; the way of having, doing, and making beings into goals, ideas, or things. What we miss is our particularity, presence, and freedom as individuals. When we are overly committed to doing, or controlling and mastering a situation, there is no space for being and true meeting. Further, and this is one of Buber's great contributions, there is no space for our integration as whole persons.

Buber offers a radically relational view of persons, one that acknowledges our dependency, wholeness, separateness, and choice. It has been a major source of inspiration, comfort, and guidance in terms of how I understand who I am and what I experience in relationships with others, including my work as a therapist. Heidegger takes us to the edge of encounter, where "the being that is me" and "the beings that are not" begin to rustle, be glimpsed, and emerge. Buber takes us into the heart of this experience; a place where selves are born:

> The You encounters me by grace—it cannot be found by seeking .... The You encounters me. But I enter into a direct relationship to it. Thus the relationship is election and electing, passive and active at once .... The concentration and fusion into a whole being can never be accomplished by me, can never be accomplished without me. I require a You to become; becoming I, I say You. All actual life is encounter .... The present—not that which is like a point ... but the actual and fulfilled present—exists only insofar as presentness, encounter, and relation exist. Only as the You becomes present does presence come into being. (Buber, 1923, p. 62)

Wholeness does not come from simply adding the parts. We are stirred or called forth into our wholeness as persons through meeting the other as an individual. This suffuses our meeting the world and becoming who we are with aliveness, unknowing, and vulnerability. Through meeting the other, our being comes into presence.

Although knowledge and techniques have all been important in my integrative journey, the decisive factor has been particular relationships and encounters. My entire whakapapa[3] of integration would be very long indeed. In the context of this chapter, certain people come to mind. These people are healers of various modalities. What they have in common is not that they work in the same technical way (they do not), or that they are people of mind, body, and spirit (who is not?), but that they were genuinely themselves with me, they allowed space for me to be who I am in the relationship with them, and they were open to the possibility of being changed through our meeting. Buber called this sort of relationship dialogue.[4]

Dialogue begins with one party turning towards the other. This happens every day, "every hour and quite trivially", when we physically turn our body towards someone else and address them, with or without words (Buber, 1947, p. 22). When we turn to the other with our "essential being", "one person steps forth and becomes a presence." (ibid., p. 25). If we are lucky, most of us know what it feels like to be with someone who is genuinely themselves, yet stands with an essential openness towards us. They do give up themselves to be with us. They let us see, however subtly, how we are with them. I remember meeting someone like this a few years ago. Our meeting lasted for about two minutes and consisted of looking into each other's eyes. Neither of us said anything, or had any clear agenda or goal. For a moment we were naked; soul-to-soul. The world was still there, with its pain, numbness, and confusion. For one moment I was reminded I had a soul; I am soul; and this other person before me is soul too. It was the briefest of meetings, but it stayed my loneliness at the time and still lives inside me to this day as a fire. Buber called this power of presence confirmation: we are confirmed as we are, and all that we potentially are as well (ibid., pp. 39–45; Hycner and Jacobs, 1995, pp. 22–25, 71–73); "In the present lies hidden what can become." (Friedman, 1985, p. 135; quoted in Hycner and Jacobs, 1995, p. 72).

While our meetings and encounters with the other may involve words, some of Buber's most moving examples are of dialogue in the presence of silence, and in the language of unspoken feeling, gesture, and touch. In the context of integrative, MindBody work, it is especially important to notice this. Whilst dialogue is often talked about as being between people, for Buber the other could be a stone or a tree, a horse, an angel, or God; "the limits of the possibility of dialogue are the limits of awareness" (Buber, 1947, p. 12). Specifically, Buber distinguished three levels of "relation": our life with nature where "the relation vibrates in the dark and remains below language"; our life with persons where "the relation is manifest and enters language ....We give and receive the You"; and our life with spiritual beings where "the relation is wrapped in a cloud", and we feel "addressed", albeit mysteriously (Buber, 1923, pp. 56–57). Through all of these spheres, "through every-thing that becomes present to us", we "gaze" towards "the eternal You; in each we perceive a breath of it; in every You we address the eternal You, in every sphere according to its manner." (ibid., p. 57).

Whoever the other is, Buber was adamant that dialogue is a concrete event. We face the other "not framed by thought but bodily present before us" (Buber, 1947, p. 32). Through encounter, we "understand in a bodily way" (ibid., p. 34).

> When I was eleven years of age, spending the summer on my grandparents' estate, I used, as often as I could do it unobserved, to steal into the stable and gently stroke the neck of my darling, a broad dapple-grey horse. It was not a casual delight but a great, certainly friendly, but also deeply stirring happening. If I am to explain it now, beginning from the still very fresh memory of my hand, I must say that what I experienced in touch with the animal was the Other, the immense otherness of the Other, which, how-ever, did not remain strange like the otherness of the ox and the ram, but rather let me draw near and touch it. When I stroked the mighty mane, sometimes marvellously smooth-combed, at other times just as astonishingly wild, and felt the life beneath my hand, it was as though the element of vitality itself bordered on my skin, something that was not I, was certainly not akin to me, palpably the other, not just another, really the Other itself; and yet it let me approach, confided itself to me, placed itself elementally in the rela-tion of *Thou* and *Thou* with me. (ibid., pp. 26–27)

There are interesting parallels between Buber's account of dialogue (above), and Merleau-Ponty's philosophy of the lived body (Merleau-Ponty, 1945; Kennedy, 2005). Both emphasize our rich, sentient inter-change in concrete engagement with the world. In the following passage David Abram explains Merleau-Ponty's theory of perception in a way that sounds distinctly like the young Buber in his grandparents' stable:

> Like the bowl, each presence [in the room] presents some facet that catches my eye while the rest of it lies hidden behind the horizon

of my current position, each one inviting me to focus my senses upon it, to let the other objects fall into the background as I enter into its particular depth. When my body thus responds to the mute solicitation of another being, that being responds in turn, disclosing to my senses some new aspect or dimension that in turn invites further exploration. By this process my sensing body gradually attunes itself to the style of this other presence—to the *way* of this stone, or tree, or table—as the other seems to adjust itself to my own style and sensitivity. In this manner the simplest thing may become a world for me, as, conversely, the thing or being comes to take its place more deeply in *my* world .... It is a sort of silent conversation that I carry on with things, a continuous dialogue that unfolds far below my verbal awareness .... (Abram, 1996, p. 52)

There are differences between Buber and Merleau-Ponty. If perception is a continuous conversation with the world, dialogue is much more fragile; much more dependent on the will of both parties, on the grace of both and beyond, and on their capacity to commit to the space between (Buber, 1923, p. 58). In the above story of Buber and the horse, the dialogue ends when Buber subtly withdraws his presence from the exquisite space between him and the horse, and thus becomes less present with the other. The horse, being exquisite, reads this and turns its presence away.

Buber often characterized dialogue as marked by genuine and unreserved communication (Buber, 1947). This does not mean blurting out anything, or simply speaking one's mind to another, although it is possible that this could happen and that a genuine meeting could still occur. Buber's comments on unreserved communication need to be read alongside what he called inclusion. That is, facing the other, being with the other, communicating back and forth in dialogue involves an inclusive presence; one capable of experiencing the other side of the dialogue while genuinely holding one's felt truth at the same time (Buber, 1947, pp. 24, 114). This was Buber's version of empathy (in a way), although empathy had too much of a selfless, disembodied flavour for Buber; it "excluded" too much of one's concreteness (ibid., p. 115). In contrast:

Inclusion ... is the extension of one's own concreteness, the fulfilment of the actual situation of life, the complete presence of the reality in which one participates. Its elements are, first, a relation, of no matter what kind, between two persons, second, an event experienced by them in common, in which at least one of them actively participates, and, third, the fact that this one person, without forfeiting anything of the felt reality of his activity, at the same time lives through the common event from the standpoint of the other ... [and comes to] understand in a bodily way ... (ibid., pp. 34, 115)

Buber's concept of inclusion is irreducibly bodied and arguably closer to our actual experience than "empathy" and "attunement" (see Staemmler, 2009). In Lynne Jacobs's words, inclusion is "a full-bodied turning-towards-the-other that includes empathy, but is more visceral than the way we usually describe empathy" (Jacobs, quoted in Staemmler, 2009, p. 78). Sometimes this happens in ways that surprise our more rigid boundary assumptions regarding body and self. On another occasion I was sitting in a group as leader. The group was just getting settled. I noticed I was feeling relaxed and solid. Everyone had found their seating and it was now time for us to begin. The group became more silent and present to each other. As we all took a moment to connect with ourselves and our sitting together, I noticed that my stomach was clenched and sore. This was surprising as I had felt quite peaceable a moment before, and, to the best of my awareness, I did not feel nervous about being in the group at that point. I became curious about whether this feeling was mine, or part of my sensitivity to the wider, present field. I decided to take a risk and ask the group.

> As I sit here I notice that my tummy is suddenly clenched and sore, which is strange as I'm not aware of otherwise feeling upset or anxious. I might be wrong, but I wonder if I'm picking up on what's in the room. Anyone else with a sore belly?

Eventually, the woman sitting beside me put up her hand. She said that her tummy was cramping and in burning pain. This was related to a current situation in her life, which she began to explore and get support from the group as she did so. As she spoke, my stomach relaxed and the soreness went away. Although this was an extraordinary experience for me, the woman, and the group; at the time it also felt normal and human. It was a risk for me to speak this way to the group, to become known in this way, and a risk for the woman to put up her hand, and make her own cramping stomach and personal suffering so known to the others too. Yet, having taken the risk, it felt like the simplest thing to do.

Earthquakes, cow country, and an intimate field

I used to think that we held back from fully experiencing and owning our own bodily experience because we had been culturally trained to think of the body as an object; irrelevant, or only marginally relevant to our richer, psychological-personal being, or self. However, as I've come to directly experience my own estrangement, mainly through my own personal therapy, and to more fully inhabit the body that is me (Merleau-Ponty, cited in Kennedy, 2005 p. 110), I have to come to see that there is something more fundamental and personal that gets in the way. For if the body is not a thing at all, but me in the flesh; me in my full richness and sensitivity; "palpably the other" in Buber's words (Buber, 1947, p. 27)—and if I require a You to become, this makes MindBody integration a radically intimate process (see also Broom, 1997, pp. 62–63). The deeper question for me, underneath our estrangement, is not so much whether I am prepared to consider my body as an expression of mind (which is still a very good question), but whether I am willing to be so sensitively, clearly, and authentically me, and be so richly, intimately known?

I would like to offer a clinical vignette of what is possible when two parties; in this case, a client and a therapist (me) are willing to be intimately known to each other (which is the true meaning of intimacy, or "intimate"—to make known, to disclose as defined …), and willing to allow the full presence of their speaking bodies to enliven the dialogue.[5]

To further emphasize the connectedness we work with, the following session occurred after the devastating Christchurch earthquakes of 2010/2011; a trauma that both the client and I, however differently, both shared and share together in our wider field of being.

> I have worked with "Toby" for almost three years. This session occurred many weeks after the violent Christchurch earthquake (called by some an "aftershock") that happened on 22 February, 2011. Toby was in a high rise building in the central city when the earthquake struck. He has been extremely anxious since then, suffering from post-traumatic stress symptoms, including feeling

in a state of high alert, startling easily at the sound of loud noises and in response to loud bangs (the many aftershocks were not helping), feeling energetically drained, feeling dizzy, suffering from constant headaches and a racing heart, sleeping extremely poorly (being unable to sleep for more than a few hours), and experiencing flashback dreams of being in the building and running through the city to pick up his children from school.

As we begin the session, I notice that Toby looks braced and cramped in his legs, arms, and torso, he looks white, drawn, and strained in his face, his breathing is erratic (held and weak at rest, quick and fast when he hears a loud car), and that he makes automatic jittery movements when he hears loud cars going by outside shaking the building. His energy feels both tired and restless. This is how he has been since the earthquake. I feel calm, solid, and caring in his presence.

Toby begins feeling angry and scattered. He is angry with his workplace. Following the first major earthquake of September 2010, on engineers' advice, they made staff return to work in the building even though it suffered considerable damage. Anger gives way to fear, and, for a few moments, Toby speaks about being in the building when the violent February earthquake struck. Toby moves quickly away from this terrifying memory. He thinks about the building instead. He has heard that it is marked for demolition. Toby begins to well up with tears. He feels sorry for the building. He imagines the building on its knees; "it's as if the building has fallen to its knees before being buried", he says.

The building is on its knees, "waiting to be put down". I ask Toby if he has any last words for the building: "I'm sorry", he says, beginning to cry, "Sorry for running out and leaving you". I see the muscles in his face and throat are working hard to hold back the tears. After a few moments I say: "Are those words just for the building?" "No", Toby says. He tells me about running out of the building, leaving others behind, and the people he saw on the streets; injured, perhaps dying, some crushed under fallen masonry. He feels guilty for not stopping to help. He ran and ran through the streets, running for his life, but most of all running to see if his children were safe. Toby is crying now. I stay silently present with him, then share my sense of how terrified and concerned he must have felt, and how in these moments his body must have wanted desperately to live, to feel safe, to get away from danger, and to be close to and protect his precious children. Toby cries heavily, bent forward and down, then comes to the end of his tears. A big sigh. I feel warm, patient, and compassionate.

Toby's head now drops to his right as he leans back in his chair very slightly. He moves his right hand so it comes to rest gently on his chest. I am moved by this simple, tender gesture. I feel a surge of warmth in my chest. I ask Toby how the hand feels. "Nice", he says after a moment, "it's soothing my heart". "What words is it saying to your heart?" I ask. "There, there. It's what I do with my kids."

Toby is much quieter now. He looks less scattered and jittery, but remains very pale, and appears cramped and flat. As I observe him, and sit in the quiet space with him, I feel tense in my muscles and have a sense of wanting to shake and stretch. I don't share this at this point; instead I am silent with him; in this I feel warm, steady, present and abiding; waiting for, but not needing, anything to happen.

Toby's head now turns and he looks to one side. His eyes lift up. He seems to have established a distant focus. I ask Toby where his attention is now. He says he is thinking of being on holiday as a boy. His Dad and he used to go on holiday to a rural part of New Zealand. I invite Toby to stay with the memory (I am slightly excited and curious; this sounds like a potentially supportive withdrawal in the present circumstances).[6]

Toby remembers being outside in the fields. The fields were full of cows. He was extremely curious about them. I remember my own curiosity about cows; my wife's parents are farmers; and how I recently discovered that cows are intensely curious creatures. I share this with Toby, and tell him about my last Christmas holiday with the in-laws, sitting at the fence looking at cows, and all the cows coming over to look at me; gazing at me for ages as they stood and chewed their grass. Toby is excited too (laughs, glows, rises in his chair, body moves forward towards me a little); he knows what I mean about the cows. He remembers sitting at a fence too, with the cows on the other side looking back at him. He remembers their rough, sticky, wet, grassy tongues. He remembers their big, loud, warm breaths. As he talks about their breathing my lungs start to expand. I see that Toby breathes in deeply too and his chest expands. I share my observations with him. He isn't aware of the breathing, but laughs and takes in a deep breath, and breaths out a big, grassy, bellow-like breath. I see that his chest opens with this breath. He looks a bit warmer in his face. I invite him to continue with the cow-style breathing, and offer to breathe in this way too. We have fun for a few moments, breathing like cows. We feel a bit awkward; neither of us has breathed like a cow before but this does not stop us trying.

As we embody the breathing cows, we start to chew grass as well; chewing and breathing like cows, just as they chew and breathe at the same time. I notice my jaw feels a little tense. This chewing feels really good for my jaw. I share that the chewing movement feels good for me, in an even way, and invite Toby to stay with the chewing too. He gets into it, chewing a little bit at first, and then developing the chewing movement into big, rolling circles of the jaw. I see that the colour in Toby's face is brighter. As I watch him chewing, chewing myself, I realize how locked his face and jaw had looked before; grim, locked like in death. Now his face is animated and moving expressively. Most of all, we are having fun.

We chew and breathe and moo a bit. I ask Toby to notice how his body is feeling. He looks interested; he says he feels much fresher and stronger in his body. He is no longer white in his face. He looks warm at present, not anxious. His body looks more muscularly relaxed; his chest is a little more open. I notice that his shoulders are in the same posture as when we began; rolled over and down, so his chest is still rounded inwards, and his tummy still collapses outwards, leaving less breathing room inside. I wonder whether to share this or not. I decide to share these observations, hoping Toby will not feel criticized. I affirm that his colour looks so much better and he is looking relaxed. I also add that I notice his shoulders are slightly rounded over. Toby is interested in this; a new piece of knowledge for him. He rolls them back, without prompting from me. His chest opens. I invite him to breathe fully again, in this position. He breathes for a few moments. His chest and belly expand and contract. Toby's body is moving; so much more mobile than how he began the session; and moving from the inside, led by his breathing and his/our warm, limbic, bovine fantasies.

Toby ends the session feeling much stronger and he looks much stronger. I feel more fresh and alive as well. Two days later, much to my surprise, Toby emails me at work to say how much he enjoyed the session, he is sleeping better, and his flashback dreams have stopped. He ends the email: "No night worries! Moo, chew, moo, chew." As the weeks pass by, this progress lasts.

I feel warmth in my belly now, as I look back on this session. I connect with the rhythm and the quality of the space; a slow, still, yet pulsing warmth, and a sense of lightness and ground in which to move, stretch, and breathe. I think about Toby and I; how we created the space between, out of our longings, swamps, and steady grounds. I connect with a sense of us, and with what can emerge when we consciously share our embodiment.

Can intimacy occur through somatic disease?

I realize that speaking of bodies and intimate fields raises many questions, including those arising around intimacy and erotic experience, which cannot be explored here but are part of the complexity we live with.

In the context of this book, focussed on the transformation of the clinician, I would like to end with some final thoughts, and with this question: Can intimacy occur through somatic disease? There is a special case of intimacy, of making oneself known, that is significant in my life and work as a therapist. Indeed, it is how I first got involved in this field, through my own somatic symptoms; an irritable bowel and a protracted glandular fever, which provided a passageway to my authentic suffering, longing, and potential. The passageway of illness brought me into contact with others. Many of these meetings were unfruitful; I was too fearful to be more explicit; I did not know how to more fully embody my truth. My clinicians were often fearful and confused as well; their own embodiments of personal truth were often too thin. I remember consulting with one medical professional who promised a holistic assessment. This consisted of taking a biomedical history of my symptoms, then asking the question "Where would you rather go on holiday: to a beach, city, or mountain valley?" before prescribing Bach flower remedies out of a standardized manual. My being was wholly untouched.

The passageway of illness also brought me into life-giving contact with the presence of others, in which my being was acknowledged, respected, and stirred. I began to learn how I embody the truth of who I am. This learning is the first step in integration and healing. This chapter is another step; a further embodiment.

Brian Broom (1997, 2000, 2002 and 2007) has written extensively on these themes; on what he calls somatic metaphor and meaning-full disease, where the body seems to express something more about a person's self and existence. Of course, this is an extremely complex and nuanced field, and a breeding ground for rash and irresponsible assumptions if one is not careful. We sometimes assign meanings in MindBody work (and generally in life) in a desperate, anxious, or rigid way. We assign rather than discover and experience our meanings. The meaning of a person's illness must be truly discovered through a genuine dialogue of what is happening (Broom, 1997). We need space to hear and hold the many voices of the dialogue (the patient's fear; the doctor's modelling; the symptom's phenomenology; the illness' onset, shape, and development; the patient's actual words to us, their story, their energy in the session; our story, our energy, life-context, fear, and modelling) and the surge of what happens when we meet.

Illness, at the very least, reveals our vulnerability, and this is always tender ground for our meetings, mergers, and separations as people. I remember visiting my mother-in-law while she was receiving chemotherapy in a very crowded hospital ward. She was vulnerable, present, and open. I got to see her and meet her more as person in that visit than at almost any other time, although the content of what we said eludes me now. I also saw and met other individuals; a businessman from somewhere, a retired farmer from somewhere else; and saw them connecting with each other, plugged into their life-prolonging drips, with an immediacy that most New Zealand men avoid, postpone, or fudge. Most of this happened in a wordless space, one that we could barely acknowledge, and yet it is the part that stays with me the most.

References

Abram, D. (1996). *The spell of the sensuous: perception and language in a more-than-human world*. New York: Vintage.

Barlow, C. (1991). *Tikanga Whakaaro: key concepts in Maori culture*. Melbourne: Oxford University Press.

Berman, M. (1989). *Coming to our senses: body and spirit in the history of the west*. London: Unwin Hyman.

Broom, B. (1997). *Somatic illness and the patient's other story: a practical integrative Mind/Body approach to disease for doctors and psychotherapists.* London: Free Association Books.
Broom, B. (2000). Medicine and story: a novel clinical panorama arising from a unitary mind/body approach to physical illness. *Advances in Mind/Body Medicine, 16:* 161–207.
Broom, B. (2002). Somatic metaphor: a clinical phenomenon pointing to a new model of disease, personhood, and physical reality. *Advances in Mind-Body Medicine, 18:* 16–29.
Broom, B. (2007). *Meaning-full Disease: How personal experience and meanings cause and maintain physical illness.* London: Karnac.
Buber, M. (1970). *I and Thou.* (Translated by Walter Kaufman). New York: Touchstone.
Buber, M. (2002). *Between man and man.* Translated by Ronald Gregor Smith. London: Routledge.
Heidegger, M. (1935). *Poetry, Language, Thought.* Translated by A. Hofstadter. New York: Harper and Row, 1971.
Hycner, R. & Jacobs, L. (1995). *The healing relationship in Gestalt therapy: a dialogic/self psychology approach.* Gouldsboro, ME: Gestalt Journal Press.
Kennedy, D. (2005). The lived body. *British Gestalt Journal, 14 (2):* pp. 109–117.
Kepner, J. (2003). The embodied field. *British Gestalt Journal, 12 (1):* pp. 43–64.
Latner, J. (1983). This is the speed of light: field and systems theories in Gestalt therapy. *The Gestalt Journal, VI (2):* pp. 71–90.
Levine, P. A. (1997). *Waking the tiger, healing trauma: the innate capacity to transform overwhelming experiences.* Berkeley, CA: North Atlantic Books.
Merleau-Ponty, M. (1945). *Phenomenology of perception.* Translated (1958) by Colin Smith. London: Routledge, 2002.
Moi, T. (1991). *The Kristeva reader.* Oxford: Blackwell.
Parlett, M. (1991). Reflections on field theory. *British Gestalt Journal, 1:* pp. 68–91.
Parlett, M. (1997). The unified field in practice. *Gestalt Review, 1 (1):* pp. 16–33.
Parlett, M. (2005). Contemporary Gestalt therapy: field theory. In: A. L. Woldt and S. M. Toman (Eds.), *Gestalt therapy: history, theory, and practice.* (pp.). Thousand Oaks, CA: Sage.
Perls, F. (1969). *Gestalt therapy verbatim.* New York: Bantam.
Smith, R. G. (1966). *Martin Buber.* London: Carey Kingsgate Press.
Staemmler, F.-M. (2009). On macaque monkeys, players, and clairvoyants: some ideas for a Gestalt therapeutic concept of empathy. In: D. Ullman &, G. Wheeler (Eds.), *CoCreating the field: Intention and practice in the age of complexity* (pp. 43–64). New York: Routledge.

Yontef, G. (1993). *Awareness, process, and dialogue: essays on Gestalt therapy.* Gouldsboro, ME: The Gestalt Journal Press.

Notes

1. In gestalt therapy we speak of the field as not just a sphere of activity ("the field of science", "the field of MindBody work"), but as the total, interconnected, contemporary situation, or the holistic present life-space of a person or a group of people, including how reality is variously experienced and known (see Latner, 1983, 1992; Parlett 1991, 1997, 2005; Kennedy, 2003; and particularly Kepner, 2003, for an emphasis on the embodied field).

2. For a brief introduction to Buber and his background, see Smith, (1966). *Martin Buber.* London: Carey Kingsgate Press. For a discussion of Martin Buber's place in gestalt therapy, see Hycner and Jacobs (1995).

3. A Māori word meaning "to lay one thing upon another", that usually gets translated as ancestry or genealogy, but goes beyond these as well: "Whakapapa is a basis for the organization of knowledge in respect of the creation and development of all things." (Barlow, 1991, p. 173).

4. Dialogue, in Buber's sense of the term, is one of the key sources for the philosophy and method of gestalt therapy (see Yontef, 1993; Hycner and Jacobs, 1995) although its ideas are more widely applicable as well.

5. The phrase "speaking bodies" is Julia Kristeva's (see Moi, 1991). Of course, dialogue is not the only path to healing and vitality. We live in a complex, intricate field. Other therapeutic dynamics present in this session might also include expressing emotion, a positive idealizing transference, empathic attunement and containment, engaging in play, and releasing frozen energy stored from traumatic experience through gentle, progressive, spontaneous movement (see Levine, 1997).

6. For Fritz Perls, withdrawal was a form of self support (Perls, 1969, p. 65; see also p. 68).

CHAPTER FOUR

Bodies in conversation

Paul Hemmingsen

Introduction

Five decades ago I was a shy, frightened boy, being raised by parents with fundamentalist Christian beliefs. Now I am a grandfather and a psychotherapist who is able to hear the familial body stories of my clients. In between these contrasting spaces a complex story of gradual transformation unfolds, leading to my current capacity as a psychotherapist who is very comfortable with bodily communication. I describe my personal journey in transforming from a conventional psychotherapy practice to one in which bodied communication becomes an acceptable norm and a rich source of therapeutic potential. I reflect upon the personal resistances arising in psychotherapists as they begin to allow the body to be more fully part of the clinical interpersonal framework.

As a small child, I used to frustrate my parents by coming into their room every morning at dawn. "Why?" they asked repeatedly. I had no answer, except that I needed to. In later life, I realized that it was my fear that God would come in the night and take them to heaven, and I would be left behind. This was a story my mother often told me, and which sermons at church constantly reinforced; God was coming to take the believers to heaven, and woe betide those left behind. But, try as I might, I could not make the required transaction with God that would give me the assurance of salvation, and the inner certainty that I would not be traumatically separated from my parents. My fear remained.

It is perhaps unsurprising that as an adult, I pursued certainty in science, and worked for some years in the field of veterinary microbiology and as a farm advisor. This was unsatisfying, and I decided to be a farmer, to prove myself as a man and to discover for myself what it was to succeed in this line of work. I was successful, and my family was able to purchase a dairy farm. This all came crashing down, some years later, when my marriage got into difficulty.

It was with considerable struggle that I attended couples' counseling, where I found myself very challenged, and shocked as I became increasingly aware of my restricted worldview. Out of this grew a hunger for greater knowledge and understanding of myself; a personal journey that culminated in further study and my finally becoming a psychotherapist. Had I known how hard and complex this learning and self-discovery was going to be, I wonder if I would ever have started it. Moving from a childhood in which I was repeatedly told that feelings were not to be trusted to the present where I trust my feeling world and use this in my interactions with others is a profound change.

Five years ago I began study in the AUT University MindBody Healthcare post-graduate programme, and another struggle ensued with my restricted world view. The struggle started like this; three months into the programme I was full of energy, reading most days, and enjoying and agreeing with Brian Broom's book *Meaning-Full Disease* (2007). Then one day, as I turned over a certain page, I found myself in the depths of a powerful resistance. The words on the page would not make sense, I wanted to avoid them and give it all up.

Dairy farmers are made of sterner stuff. They don't give up. Come flood, come drought, they box on. I would not give up, because I wanted to understand my own reaction and resistance to what was being suggested about bodied responses. My psychotherapy supervisor of that time, Wilson Daniel, was able to hold me in this struggle about my body, my illnesses, and their meanings. This material I was reading was not just about other people, but also about me.

One example was my ongoing "farmers back." This began when I was fighting with a large round hay bale on a bad day, as the rain poured down and the cows stirred up mud. It was my first winter milking a large herd and I was desperate to prove myself, but also afraid that I would not be able to do it. I fought in a desperate and angry way with this monster bale which was stuck in a feeder, and I fought with the fear of being physically inadequate. I injured my back.

As I worked through my resistance, gradually gaining insight and understanding, I also started to notice and study my body's responses in the therapy room with psychotherapy clients. These responses began to surprise and intrigue me, and were loudest in the first session with a new client.

Here is an example from my current therapy practice.

> John is a middle-aged Maori with a very violent history. He attends at the request of his wife who has made the therapy a condition of continuing with the relationship. The first task we negotiate is how we will manage his violent urges should they arise in the therapy room. A strategy is agreed between us. Later as he begins to talk about his daily life I have tingling in my legs and a rising tightness in my chest. I ask him if he notices his body is changing. He takes his time, but says, yes, something is happening in his legs and his chest and what is this? I explain that to me it feels like fear. "Really" he says, "no one has ever told me that I am afraid, I have never thought of myself as being afraid of anyone but my body is like this most of the time. Boy that is really something." This was the start of a productive therapy process. Whenever I detected this bodied fear response I talked about it with him. This has made the therapy safe for both of us. The therapy has brought about major changes in his life.

This type of interaction did not occur in my therapy practice until I worked through the resistance that I became aware of while reading Broom's book. What is the nature of this change in me? By this I mean, why am I now aware of my physiological responses and their meanings? As the therapy began with John he experienced a physiological change; this evoked a change in me, which I then linked to his suppressed experience of fear. He has lived in a world of either being violent or experiencing others as being violent to him. His childhood had pre-disposed him to suppress his fear. Later in the therapy I learned that his father would severely physically assault him if he showed any fear or pain.

My parents are Open Brethren Christians; they believe that Jesus is about to return to the earth at any moment and take the Believers back to heaven. This would leave all the non-Believers on earth to face the Great Tribulation (a time of war and great suffering). As a child, I had to believe that my confession of faith to God would guarantee that when he took the Believers to heaven I would go as well. I had to believe to become a Believer. The reward for believing was that my terror would be gone and this would prove that the transaction with God was complete. With this assurance I could be certain that I would not be traumatically separated from my parents. I know now that I suppressed this fear, though my regular morning wakening of my parents shows the suppression was not successful. Suppression of my fear gave me a lot of secondary gain; my parents were very proud of my faith and held me up to others as an example of what a good believing boy I was. This should have assured me, but it did not. No matter how much I prayed to God, the fear did not go away.

This illuminated both my resistance to Broom's book and my previous suppression of what was happening in my body. In the vignette concerning John, we have two men whose backgrounds have predisposed them to suppress their fear. Now that I have worked though my own fear and denial of my body as a source of knowing, I can sit with John and calmly talk about our mutual physiological arousal and discover its meaning. We have both been predisposed to fear, John from a violent childhood, and me from fear of abandonment by my parents.

I have freely used the concept of suppression without providing an explanation as to exactly what I mean by this. When strong emotions emerge, along with their autonomic nervous system elements, the options are either to plan and take protective action, or to suppress the expression of this strong physical arousal, and appear calm. The latter is called expressive suppression (Richards & Gross, 2006) a form of emotional regulation. It is suggested that this comes at an emotional and cognitive cost. John and Gross (2004) propose a process model of emotional regulation. A triggering event begins a process, which can be contained by having a plan before the physiological response occurs, or the resultant feeling can be suppressed. These authors distinguish between antecedent-focused and response-focused emotional regulation. They demonstrate that intervening in emotional generation before the emotional responses have become active is healthy, compared with suppressing the expression of the emotional response after it has developed.

Amstadter (2008) discusses and reviews this model of emotional regulation in relation to anxiety disorders. He points out that in Post Traumatic Stress Disorder (PTSD) the regularity of suppression is proportional to the severity of the symptoms and that suppression of both positive and negative emotions takes place. They also conjecture that suppression may maintain the symptoms of PTSD by increasing the physiological arousal and its associated global anxiety.

Applying this to the vignette, we have John, who is suppressing his expression of fear because of his previous aversive experiences of violence when he was a child, and Paul (myself) who is suppressing because of childhood fears of abandonment. I appear to experience the physiological reaction in John, which, in contrast to John, I recognize and understand. I established this with John; we find we are experiencing the same thing and I explain it to him. He recognizes the truth of it for him. The question remains however; how does my body know what John's body is communicating?

Orbach (2009) describes how Italian neuroscientists Rizzolatti and Gallese discovered the mirror neuron system. They were tracking the firing of brain cells in monkeys, using functional MRI, as the monkeys stretched out their arms to reach for a peanut. One day an associate researcher from another laboratory came in and ate one of the peanuts and was seen doing this by one of the experimental monkeys. The researchers were astonished to find that the same cells fired up (as seen on the MRI) when the monkey saw the peanut being picked up as when the monkey actually performed the task itself. These extraordinary and unexpected results implied that the monkey brain mirrored the movements that the monkey observed.

Many experiments later (Gallese, 2006), the mirror neuron system was identified in both monkey and human brains (Rizzola and Craighead, 2004). When we observe actions, this system fires as if we are actually performing them. To put it another way, seeing is mapped onto the motor neuron system when we observe another person. This implies that the physiological arousal of a person who is suppressing their emotions cannot really be kept private. Another person can experience them physically, via the mirror neuron system. De Gelder, Synder, Greve, Gerad and Hadjikani (2004) discuss this and experiment with the idea of a fear contagion, where a brain/body experiences a fear response to another's fear. What I am attempting to show here is that there are neural mechanisms that may explain the physiological arousal that I feel sitting with John. This is a plausible explanation of why I can experience his fearful physical arousal when John seems to have no conscious awareness that he is afraid.

The way into a patient's world for most psychotherapists is through talking; through words exchanged between therapist and client, from the top down, from the conscious to the unconscious. Progress is through insight, understanding and interpretation of the transference. However, with John, I have entered into his world of experience and meaning through our joint physical experience. The Hakomi theorists Ogden and Minton (2000) call this interaction bottom-up processing. They assert that traditional psychotherapy addresses the cognitive and emotional elements of trauma but lacks the capacity to work with the physiological arousal. If we also add the observations of Amstader (2008), that suppression limits cognition and hides the expression of emotion; then this is indeed a big limitation of the psychotherapeutic method when treating autonomic nervous system arousal and Post-Traumatic Stress Disorder. Ogden and Minton use the term Sensorimotor Psychotherapy for an approach that involves top-down and bottom-up processing. In this approach the changes in the body of the client are carefully observed, and the therapist provides an auxiliary cortex to assist the client in understanding the changes within the client's body. What I am discussing and demonstrating here is the additional use not just of the cortex of the therapist but also the changes within the body of the therapist; an auxiliary body as well as an auxiliary mind to enter and understand the world of the client.

> Daniel is a man in his mid-thirties who I saw for forty sessions of therapy about eight years ago. The therapy seemed to be successful, in that he was able to finish his university degree and stabilize his social world. It ended mutually, with Daniel expressing gratitude for the help he had received. This was before my training in the MindBody approach, and before the changes in me following the resolution of my resistance. I had moved from suppressing my fears to being comfortable feeling and thinking about physiological changes in my body.
>
> Recently Daniel presented again following several years of drug abuse, which he has recently withdrawn from. The striking element

we became aware of this time was his chronic Post-Traumatic Stress Disorder relating to a serious sexual assault when he was twelve years old. He did speak of this incident in the first therapy, but said that the perpetrator had been caught and punished and that he felt fine about it. In the recent therapy, he again said that the incident had occurred and that he had come to terms with it and did not see any reason to talk about it. However, this time I had a large physiological response. I had tingling in my arms and a strong sensation in my gut. So I said to him that there was a bodied conversation occurring. "What do you mean?" he asked. I asked him to reflect on what was changing in his body and I rubbed my stomach. He responded by saying that he didn't want to talk about it. I told him that our bodies were conversing.

When he returned the next week he told me of the turmoil he had experienced during the week, because he both wanted help but wanted to keep all that his body experienced hidden. What followed was a slow unfolding of the impact of this assault on him. These interactions regularly began with strong physiological sensations that could then be thought about. An example is his description of being asked by the Police to leave a bar because he was looking angry. "I was", he said, "but I would not hurt anyone." However, they insisted and he resisted, and was given the option to leave willingly or be handcuffed. "I took the wise option and left with no drama." At this point my chest and stomach had a strong sensation, so I asked if his body was changing. He nodded and talked of his stomach being in knots. I responded by saying that it seemed to provoke a large bodily response when his arms were restrained. He nodded and tears flowed freely. After a while, he explained the intense fear that he had experienced with me. Daniel is a tall man with a confident physical bearing, who shows no sign of fear. There is a pattern to these interactions. Daniel suppresses feeling by telling me in an emotionless way about his world. My body responds to his physiological arousal which, when I put this to him in words, opens his experience up for thinking.

At the risk of being harsh on myself, I think that in the first therapy I colluded with Daniel in avoiding intense fear. Neither of us had the capacity to interact in a way that involved reflection on our physiological responses. Both of us suppressed our fear experiences, because of early life traumas and defensive patterns emerging from those. When he presented for a second therapy I had changed. I had faced my child-hood terror and through the MindBody training had gained a confi-dence in using my body to understand the world of my clients, from the bottom up. This second therapy with Daniel utilized all the usual psychotherapeutic elements relating to transference and insight, along with the physiological interactions.

In my therapy room, there are bodied conversations, especially with the group of clients who meet the criteria for PTSD and who sup-press the expression of autonomic system arousal. Somatic phenomena within therapists are widely reported (Arnold, Clahoun, Tedeschi and Cann, 2005; Stone, 2006; King, 2011). Shaw's grounded theory study of psychotherapist's somatic experiences "revealed the importance of the therapist's body within the therapeutic encounter" (2004, p. 271). This study however did not examine the responses of the client within the therapy. In the examples of John and Daniel, I was careful not to assume that their bodied responses were going to be similar to mine. There is an order to my interventions. I notice the change in my body; I then enquire if the client notices any change, and then if there is common bodily experience I lead an exploration of the phenomena. Shaw sug-gests this same order of investigation; to ask the client what is occurring in their body when there are moments of somatic resonance.

Above, I wrote about healthy, antecedent responses to autonomic triggering or unhealthy, expressive suppression later in the response path. It is clearly helpful to get the client to shift from expressive sup-pression as a defense against strong feeling, to the more open possibili-ties of the thoughtfulness of antecedent responses.

> Margaret is a woman in her early fifties who was referred to me in considerable distress with suicidal ideation. She had been a suc-cessful businesswoman, but something had happened that had traumatically disrupted her world. Slowly she explained that for as long as she could remember she had lived with an obsessive/compulsive disorder (OCD), which in some ways had helped her function. Recently this system had broken under the intense strain of an abusive work environment. Now without this way of keeping her intense feelings under control, they were overwhelming her. She was flooded with intense fear, anger and sadness; she could not cope with day-to-day life. Her defenses against her feelings had

been overwhelmed by events in her work place. Margaret has a history of multiple sexual assault and intrusion in her early life, which had recently returned to her awareness in the form of intense flashbacks. Previously she had succeeded despite the abuse, albeit with the disability of OCD. Now this method of coping was broken.

There was intense physical arousal and distress in the room. I would put my physiological resonance with this into words. The feeling would be understood and then an exploration of what was triggering it attempted. Often, Margaret would then describe an intense memory as the feeling and physical arousal were contained. This would help establish a healthy order, in contrast to the tyrannical unhealthy order of OCD, formed by linking the triggering event and the memory that was associated with it, in a calming and containing environment. She explained that it was like being with a farmer who was making calm sense of chaos. To her, it was as if the cows had got out onto the road; there was danger. I was firmly putting them back into the paddock and then repairing the broken fence. My capacity to sit calmly with her intense fear, to be an auxiliary body in a purely physical sense, was an important part of the therapy. In this way she has been able to focus on antecedent responses to her autonomic triggers. Recently she was thrown back into attempts to use the OCD as a defense. She felt that a stranger had unexpectedly invaded her personal space. When she came to the next session I felt very uncomfortable and I struggled to sit still. I wondered with her about her body sensations, which were similar to what I was experiencing. She reflected on this, and her disappointment at being back into OCD was both discussed and normalized; it will of course happen occasionally. I should add that when I was a farmer, and in my early years as a psychotherapist, I did not have the capacity to sit with these strong feelings. This capacity developed out of working with my own resistance to my body experience during the MindBody course. The therapy with Margaret lasted a few years and has been very successful, with her only occasionally resorting to the use of OCD defenses.

In this Chapter, I have discussed my personal change from a frightened boy, to a science graduate, to dairy farmer, to psychotherapist and then a body-orientated psychotherapist. The crucial change for me arose during the MindBody training, through being confronted by the need to include my body in the clinical space.

Expressive suppression, in its different guises, has been highlighted as an explanation for shared physical arousal between the therapist and client. John showed this with his extreme violence to others. Daniel resorted to an impassive manner. Margaret did not use expressive suppression, but instead OCD to avoid her feelings. There are many other potential ways in which a person as a body brings "the intimate imprint of the familial body story" (Orbach, 2009, p. 57) into the therapy room. What I have attempted to show is that shared body experience can provide helpful insight into the world of the client, provided the therapist is comfortable to sit with and think about the physical discomfort in his or her own body.

References

Amstadter, A. (2008). Emotional regulation and anxiety disorders. *Journal of Anxiety Disorders*, 22: 211–221.

Arnold, D., Clahoun, L. G., Tedeschi, R. & Cann, A. (2005). Vicarious posttraumatic growth in psychotherapy. *Journal of Humanistic Psychology, 45*: 239–263.

Broom, B. (2007). *Meaning-full disease.* London: Karnac.

De Gelder, B., Synder, J., Greve, D., Gerad, G. & Hadjikani, N. (2004). Fear fosters flight: A mechanism for fear contagion when perceiving emotion expressed by a whole body. *Proceedings of the National Academy of Science, 101(47)*: 16701–16706.

Gallese, V. (2007). Before and below 'theory of mind': Embodied simulation and the neural correlates of social cognition. *Philosophical Transactions of the Royal Society, 362*: 659–669.

John, O. & Gross, J. (2004). Healthy and unhealthy emotional regulation: Personality processes, individual differences, and life span development. *Journal of Personality, 72(6)*: 1301–1333.

King, A. (2011). When the body speaks: Tummy rumblings in the therapeutic encounter. *British Journal of Psychotherapy, 27(2)*: 156–174.

Ogden, P. & Minton, K. (2000). Sensorimotor psychotherapy: One method for processing traumatic memory. *Traumatology, 6*: 149.

Orbach, S. (2009). *Bodies.* London: Profile Books.

Richards, J. & Gross, J. (2006). Personality and emotional memory: How regulation impairs memory for emotional events. *Journal of Research in Personality, 40*: 631–651.

Rizzolatti, G. & Craighead, L. (2004). The mirror-neuron system. *Annual Review of Neuroscience 27*: 169–182.

Shaw, R. (2004). The embodied psychotherapist: An exploration of the therapists' somatic phenomena within the therapeutic encounter. *Psychotherapy Research, 14(3)*: 271–288.

Stone, M. (2006). The analyst's body as tuning fork: Embodied resonance in countertransference. *Journal of Analytical Psychology, 51*: 109–124.

CHAPTER FIVE

The proof is in the pudding

Emma Harris

Introduction

An integrative MindBody approach to healing works through the containment of the whole of the person. By using the word MindBody I am already expressing some of what it is to practise according to this philosophy. By deliberately putting mind and body together, an oppositional pull is created to separate them. My computer spell-check underlines the word MindBody in red and helpfully tells me I need to put a split down the middle, making it into two autonomous words. Grosz (1994) might argue, however, that dichotomous thinking does not allow for autonomy; rather body becomes what mind is not and therefore body is seen as subordinated to the privileged position the mind holds.

Certainly this is reflected in psychotherapy clinical practice. As a psychotherapist, I used to see my role as working with the mind, leaving the medical profession to work with the body. This norm has been tacitly engrained in Western society since Descartes' (1641) philosophy of dualism, between mind and body, commonly known as the Cartesian split. It takes effort to do something different and treat the whole of the person, because it rebels against the status quo. However, effort is only part of the equation. I believe it is the transformation of the practitioner from a dualistic position to one that can uphold a unitary framework that is crucial. This transformation creates the space and holding for the wholeness of the client to be privileged and, in turn, for healing to take place.

This Chapter reflects my own journey of integrating a MindBody philosophy into my psychotherapy practice. I describe the challenges I have faced and illustrate this developmental process with some clinical vignettes. Whilst I do not specifically address the notion of spirituality in this piece I hope the reader gains a sense that it is intrinsically there. Honouring the transpersonal relationship, and the use of mindfulness and reverie, is to me the essence of what works in psychotherapy.

In the beginning—intuition

Within my family the authority of the medical paradigm was unchallenged. "Doctorliness" was next to Godliness; it was always a case of "the Doctor said". That was the end of it because the truth had been spoken. However, being much more the kind of person who from a young age was interested in the grey-in-between, rather than the black-and-white, I never felt comfortable with the way the body was treated so separately from the mind or spirit. I remember my mother taking me to the Doctor at age twelve with severe stomach pain. I knew the real reason I was in physical pain was because I was in pain emotionally due to bullying by a peer at school. Yet perhaps because of my age I was not willing to admit to this and, as I was not asked how I felt other than physically, I did not tell them.

This example highlights the contextual importance that familial patterns and roles have in working with illness and disease. These can create very complex reasons for not wanting to address what really might be going on, just as was the case in my own family. Both McDougall (1989) and Broom (1997) imply that illness and disease can provide a kind of lifeline, which becomes so familiar the person cannot imagine life without it. Similarly the family may be unconsciously resistant to change because this may mean difficult issues and emotions, which may threaten the status quo, might have to be addressed within the family system.

As a young woman working and travelling in Europe I observed these same phenomena whilst working as a nanny. I noticed that some children would take to their sick beds when one (most often the mother) or both of their parents were about to go away on a trip without them. It seemed clear to me that the mystery illness was an expression of separation anxiety, an attachment issue rather than a medical one. One young girl, Charlotte, who I often nursed in her mother's absence, would somatize with severe migraines and nausea. After observing a pattern with these symptoms I wondered aloud to the mother whether it might not be a physical complaint, but rather an expression of how much her daughter was missing her. It was perhaps not surprising my expertise on such things as an unqualified nanny was considered less valuable than the country's top neuro-surgeon and gastroenterologist who had been consulted to find the solution to Charlotte's condition. Unsurprisingly, despite extensive scans and tests, neither could find a physical cause for her symptoms, and the status quo in the family, which felt threatened by direct identification and expression of separation anxiety, prevailed.

On one level I intuitively knew through my experiences that emotions and somatic complaints were connected but this was given little conscious thought by me at that time. It was not until I returned to New Zealand after living and working extensively in Europe, Asia and Australia for five years that I began a more academic journey. My decision to study sociology was partly influenced by my desire to make some theoretical sense of my overseas experiences. Understanding different societies through a variety of theoretical lenses taught me how to critique norms I had never consciously questioned. I was particularly drawn to post-structuralism, which for me was a bit like the difference between admiring a flower and then re-examining it through a kaleidoscope. What is initially accepted as a flower and a thing in itself becomes transformed into a complex myriad of shifting, abstract shapes and colours that provokes questions about what is being seen. This analogy illustrates the conflict I faced being ensconced in such a theoretical domain. By deconstructing norms there was a danger of losing the ability to hold onto the whole, the sum of the parts that we all present to each other, contained as we are within our bodies.

During those years at university the majority of lectures were unsurprisingly heavily theoretical. Interestingly, the few that still hold significance for me are those that were given by Maori guest speakers. Something was brought alive for me in listening to them. Instead of espousing the theories of long dead philosophers, they talked about their long dead ancestors as if they were alive for them. They spoke of the land as an integral foundation to their sense of wellbeing as a people. They bridged some gap for me between theory and practice. In other words these speakers were not reducing themselves into ever greater splits and micro-parts but rather galvanizing their wholeness by being inclusive of their minds, bodies and souls; their past, present and future. The unquestioning acceptance of the wholeness of a person that was embodied by these speakers resonated deeply with my own experience and belief system; and was stored away in a recess of my mind for future reference.

My personal quest for self-understanding and the healing of my own emotional wounds led me to engage in the process of my own therapy. Over time I experienced a more cohesive sense of self, born out of being held emotionally in a relationship. This was one of the catalysts for my decision to train as a psychotherapist. Over five years I felt as if I had moved from a macro, external perspective toward the internal, micro workings of the human psyche; and this is where I felt most comfortable. I assumed I would graduate from my studies as a holistic practitioner and that this would be fully supported by the training I undertook. However as these assumptions were not fully conscious I did not recognise what was missing for me from the course until I had completed it and begun my clinical work.

Suddenly I was faced with many clients in physical pain and chronic suffering. My very first client in my first job out of training suffered from crippling arthritis, a condition that began the day after her engagement to marry. I had little idea how to respond to this story, what to do with it, if anything. Was I, as a psychotherapist even allowed to? I will return to this question below.

Conflicting theories?

As I have suggested, my ideas and beliefs about holistic practice were still in infancy during my psychotherapy training, as personal self reflection and clinical understandings were brought deliberately to the fore. The use of Freudian theory to understand the mind by separating it into the different functions of the id, ego and super ego was helpful from a psychoanalytic perspective. However this compartmentalization of the mind tacitly reinforced the position of mind over body. It felt then that my training in psychotherapy further privileged the status quo of the

Cartesian split. It was not on my conscious radar to question this norm. My belief is that this split, implicit in psychotherapy training, stems from the inability of psychoanalysis to understand a somatic symptom as an expression of the whole person. In other words as a profession it has fundamentally left organic illness to the medical fraternity, upholding and entrenching the Cartesian split further (Bakal, 1999).

The dualistic nature of the status quo is often covert. I have experienced many settings where experienced psychotherapists have been comfortable talking about their clients' illnesses or disease; but only if that illness could be neatly framed as a direct reflection of what was occurring in the unconscious. The problem would remain because this is where the thinking ended. In other words, the mind and body might conveniently be stitched together when a common thread was identified but the rest of the time they remained separate. This stitching together acts like a temporary tacking up of a loose hem; it works for the moment but sooner or later will once again come undone. I believe this is because the body feels in a way tacked on to many types of psychotherapy rather than it being an inclusive and integral part of the practitioner's practice.

For example, much of my psychotherapy training involved self-reflection, awareness, emotional congruence and the ability to be aware of my own prejudices and learning edges. The same was not true of the stories of my body and spirit or how I viewed them in relation to my mind. I was not made aware of my unconscious dualistic beliefs about the mind and body. I believe until a practitioner is able to know these edges in themselves, the ability to work from a holistic philosophy will be compromised and ineffectual for the client.

Maybe we need to look back to last century to the work of clinicians such as Georg Groddeck to gain a more inclusive perspective. Groddeck firmly believed the distinctions between mind and body to be verbal constructs and he offered a restoration of Freud's more deconstructive methods of analysis. The passage below reflects the perfect symbiotic nature of the origins of human life, a relationship we yearn for on some level in our consciousness for the rest of our lives. Groddeck's insight into the human condition is eloquent and deeply perceptive.

> Never again in his life does the human being have relations as intimate as those that he entertains with his mother during pregnancy. The extent to which we harbour the wish to love and be loved is

> conditioned by this period of most intimate togetherness. The It
> in us retains the memory of perfect togetherness and urges and
> seeks a repetition, breaks up the unified love of the child into a
> thousand ever-changing parts which are being transferred to peo-
> ple, animals, plants, dead and living objects, ideas and creations,
> and now and then they produce larger emotional complexes.
> (Groddeck, 1997, p. 138)

The significance of this first, core intimate experience in the womb is
not to be underestimated for the integral influence it has on our intimate relationships. Awareness of our own MindBody origins and histories as well as those of our clients, lays a strong foundation at the
beginning of the work.

> For example, Lily, a client who suffered from crippling migraines
> for many years would take to her bed for days. She would tell me
> "the headaches and painkillers are like a blanket that muffle out
> the world." Lily began life as a premature baby who spent her first
> weeks in an incubator. We worked out over time that it felt safer for
> her to have a migraine than have to deal with her feelings and terror
> of being attached, firstly to her mother and then to me. During that
> time I had to sit with my own discomfort and uncertainty as she
> continued to embody physical pain rather than face the emotional
> risk of trusting me. For many months I felt I was sitting beside that
> incubator trying to make contact through a wall of plastic. I had to
> be patient for a long time before Lily felt able to connect with me,
> her feelings of attachment, and the world. Only when Lily allowed
> herself to feel did the migraines begin to dissipate.

The inclusive nature of this approach contrasts sharply with the biomedical discourse in Western society which often further fragments a
person's sense of unity and wholeness. What is instead valued is scientific evidence that is gleaned from clinical trials that require participants
to fit neatly into pre-determined criteria in order to be able to gener-
alise findings to the whole population. This perpetuates an on-going
reductionist ideology that fails to address the core of each person's
uniqueness. The holism of a person becomes reduced to a set of parts,
disconnected and out of touch with the other, both intra-psychically
and interpersonally. It seems to me unsurprising that some of the most
common clinical issues people bring to my psychotherapy practice are
those of addiction, depression (including post-natal depression) and

anxiety. Alternatively they may come with a physical complaint such as obesity, anorexia or chronic physical illness. These clients often describe an overwhelming sense of emptiness. I believe society perpetuates this emptiness through its pre-occupation with the external, exacerbated by the growth industry of appearance medicine and targeting treatment of specific bodily areas rather than the whole person.

So what is to be done? It is my belief that we need to re-focus our direction in working with illness. What has been concentrated on in the twenty-first century is the analysis and deconstruction of the mind and body; perhaps without much thought for how we can restore our fragmented selves. My philosophy of MindBody psychotherapy has containment at its core. The whole person needs to be held in mind and feel contained because, like an ecosystem, you cannot change one aspect in isolation without the rest of the system being affected.

What makes MindBody therapy effective is, as I stated at the beginning of this Chapter, the transformation of the therapist. Groddeck proposed that the clinician needed to practise with the belief that "nothing human is strange to me" (1997, p. 1). This statement suggests an almost tangible holding of the client, inviting them to bring themselves fully and wholly to the work. Additionally and perhaps conversely I believe it is my job as a clinician to also see everything as strange, in order to be curious and interested in understanding what may be happening for the client, myself, and our relationship. Most importantly I need to attend to myself in order to be with another. This has been about valuing the depth and breadth of my own strangeness so I can be more aware of what belongs to me rather than my client. In this regard one's own therapy and supervision can provide essential insight and awareness to one's own blind spots as well as providing containment and holding for the client.

Early on, some of my blind spots had to do with not understanding what covert ideologies underpin the nature of psychotherapy; and with the academic belief in the Cartesian split, which I was unaware I carried with me. Over time I have identified that working as a psychotherapist gave me less authority in contrast to a profession that fully embraced the bio-medical framework. This is symbolic of positivist ideology at work. As psychotherapeutic enquiry does not lend itself to the standardized measurement used to inform evidence-based medicine and practice, I perceived its method as less valid or legitimate based on my own medical upbringing. Psychotherapy faces a challenge to produce evidence because its method relies much more on spontaneous responses that reflect the unique relational dynamics between therapist and client.

So it might be said that in the hierarchy of the New Zealand health-care system, psychotherapy already has a quiet voice. This is then over-laid by the supposedly controversial idea that the body can be worked with and healed through a process of talking. Further complicating this already unlikely scenario is that it seems virtually impossible to really measure and quantify how this happens. In this regard, I agree with Mehl-Madrona's assertion that attempts to quantify and/or qualify these interventions can inadvertently destroy the delicacy of the rela-tional field that heals. He asks "How can we do research when the mere attempt at measurement, or even the intent to measure, could destroy the phenomena?" (2005, p. 18). The delicacy of the relational field reflects the uniqueness of the intersubjective relationship between the therapist and client rather than a generic recipe. It relies on ingredients from each of our unique stories, historical context and attachments, and how those are played out through the relational dynamics between the client and therapist. The measurement is how the person feels during and at the end of the process; in other words, the proof is in the pudding.

A further differentiation between the medical model and psycho-therapy is the concept of doing as opposed to being. My first efforts at MindBody therapy with clients were very much about doing, in other words technique-driven and overt. By MindBody therapy I mean utiliz-ing psychotherapeutic technique to widen the framework to allow the whole person in the room. However, as I have discovered, this allowing is a process and personally I needed to face an uncomfortable sense of lack before I could begin to engage with a different way of being. Only then could I have faith in the notion that the clinical relationship was actually capable of facilitating healing of illness or disease with a treat-ment plan that primarily puts intangible qualities such as faith, hope, love and care in the core of the process.

During this time I was surprised at my own resistance and the strength of my unconscious privileging of the bio-medical model over a more integrative way of working. Whilst I consciously believed in an integrative approach to working with somatic illness, I struggled to hold what I knew, in the room, with the clients I was seeing. The tacit dualistic beliefs I had grown up with were hard to shake off. This was particularly so with clients I saw early on who were very medical-ized. I realised that the dualistic split between mind and body can be a present and powerful unconscious dynamic in the room. The following case example illustrates the difficulties I was presented with, both for myself intra-psychically and with the client interpersonally.

> Penny, a young client, came to see me for psychoanalytic psycho-therapy to deal with emotional distress arising from an unstable relationship with her boyfriend, resulting in Penny feeling suicidal. Penny and I quickly established a good rapport and she was able to connect to ambivalent feelings toward her boyfriend. About half way through the ten sessions she mentioned in passing she had had a chronic urinary tract infection. This had begun after they first began a sexual relationship and was continually exacerbated by sexual intercourse. I felt posed with a dilemma; Penny had come to me for psychological help yet it also seemed to me that her body was expressing the ambivalence she felt toward her boyfriend through a physical infection.
>
> Clearly there were many emotional levels Penny and I could work through concerning her developing identity and processes around separation and individuation she was experiencing. Yet whilst Penny used the mind therapy effectively, there was little freedom between us to address the idea that the urinary infection was not just a physical complaint. Any attempt by me to reflect on the parallels between what her mind and body might be expressing felt somewhat artificial compared with my usual psychotherapeu-tic way of relating, and created more distance between Penny and I. Penny would then repeat her decision that she planned to take her doctor's advice and continue taking the three months worth of antibiotics, despite them having no positive impact to date. My response was to also move away from trying to contain Penny's body in the therapy, feeling it much easier to leave her GP to deal with it. I could not contain the split that was invariably there and instead continued to focus on Penny's emotional needs. Penny left therapy after ten sessions feeling much stronger emotionally, but her physical infection remained unchanged.

This example highlights the importance in recognizing one's own split off dimensions as a practitioner. Could Penny really embrace her wholeness if I was unable to integrate my own? The unconscious obstacles to fully maintaining a MindBody stance with Penny had a number of contextual layers that presented themselves in the mix of the inter-subjective relationship. The Cartesian split between mind and body was overt in Penny and covert in me. Her belief that her GP would take care of her body and I would take care of her mind was embedded as the norm; it was both hard to recognize and hard to change. I felt my professional knowledge becoming subordinated by the norms of the bio-medical status quo. I call it unconscious positivism.

In addition, there was a non-verbal layer of communication between Penny and myself. According to McDougall (1989), somatic presentation is the representation of something previously unable to be verbalized and directly correlates with some disturbance in a relational capacity. The disturbance that was enacted between Penny and I was the dynamic of "acting upon" rather than "being with," a familiar theme in Penny's story. In my need for Penny to understand what I believed her body to be expressing I acted as an authority without leaving her space to find her truth for herself.

Using the loose hem analogy, I had unwittingly stitched a set of theories onto my usual way of working. Having not yet successfully integrated a MindBody perspective into my practice, I instead acted out Grosz's (1994) statement on dichotomous thinking by privileging MindBody theory, and I let the relational way in which I normally work become subordinated. Ironically this process of "acting upon" was more reflective of the biomedical paradigm than a MindBody one.

Hope and change

I have come to understand that metabolizing a shift in thinking into a state of being is a process that takes time. Supporting oneself with reading the work by others from a variety of disciplines and historical times is essential in facilitating this shift. Winnicott is one theorist and clinician who conveys the essence of what it is to be whole. He explains the "I am" as the ability "to achieve a unity of the psyche and the soma, an experiential identity of the spirit or psyche and the totality of physical functioning" (1966, p. 514). He later describes this as the "indwelling of the psyche in the soma" (p. 515) in which the whole person can then enjoy psychosomatic unity.

Ken Wilber's (2000) exhaustive research into what he calls the four faces of the cosmos have been useful for examining the depth and breadth of an individual's unique story, my own as well as my clients.

He provides a framework that brings to consciousness possible aspects of one's own unconscious dimensions. This is largely because of the inclusiveness of Wilber's model. He addresses not just the individual's interior and exterior world (feelings, emotions, thoughts and the body's physical sensations through the skin, cells and tissue) but also the internal workings of collective beliefs. This includes elements such as the worldview, values and beliefs of cultures and commonality of shared experiences, as well as the exterior of the collective such as social structures, family dynamics and systems. His model reminds me of the imagery and story told in the existentialist film "The Tree of Life" (2011). Director Terrence Malick uses contrasting imagery reflective of all aspects of life from the pre-historic to intrauterine to the cosmos. It highlights the significance that all our experiences, whether known or remembered, contribute in some way to who we are as people.

By engaging in an on-going process of seeking self-knowledge and awareness one can develop and work from a new set of integrative beliefs. These beliefs can manifest as increased internal emotional space, trust, faith and hope. In other words, the resulting internal spaciousness within me as the clinician can then aid my attunement to what the client is trying to communicate to me. In my own experience those clients that get better do so because they feel contained in the therapeutic relationship. Containment includes the aforementioned elements of trust, hope, and faith but also holds a holistic framework that welcomes the wholeness of the person. It is about not expecting a client to leave his or her body at the door but having an inclusive we-can-deal-with-all-of-you attitude when they arrive.

When one's whole being can be used in the relationship with another, one can then "serve" as opposed to "treat" one's clients. According to Groddeck, "treating" a person is a conscious process whereby the practitioner uses their knowledge and ability to do so. In contrast, "serving" a patient requires one's "whole being, in other words the whole of his conscious and unconscious being" (1977, p. 211). He points out that as the unconscious is outside one's own intentionality its usefulness can only lie in its effects rather than as an intentional form of treatment. Hence the on-going reflection through supervision of what those effects might be.

The following case example returns to the story of my client who suffered from arthritis and illustrates a moment in our work in which a transformation of consciousness took place.

In a session early on in our work Diana (who suffered from a crippling generalized arthritis) explained that that day was the anniversary of her mother's death. Quickly she gulped and swallowed hard, interrupting any potential flow of tears that immediately filled her eyes. She changed the subject to talk about having to "put things in boxes" at work. In response I felt simultaneously as though I had an object like a box lodged in my stomach that I wanted desperately to dispel through wailing or shouting.

I reflected to Diana my sense of how hard it might be for her to just let the tears come. Diana looked relieved telling me she was feeling a very familiar blockage in her throat "It is my warning sign and it stops the tears ... and reminds me to pull myself together." Diana then remembered how she received the message from her father not to be "weak and emotional" by overtly being told to "pull yourself together." She then acknowledged: "I needed to protect my father from my grief, he needed me to be strong for him." I could then bring the possibility that she might also need to protect me from her grief in that moment, effectively trying to unconsciously put her emotions and feelings in a box. Her recognition of what was happening between us was palpable in the moment and in hindsight pivotal for the laying down of trust in our relationship and for many tears to come as she gradually allowed expression of her feelings.

I believe the wholeness of our two beings connected with one another in that moment in a way that was mutually transformative. This was a moment of healing. Over time Diana's arthritis improved to the point she stopped all but one of the many medications she was on and told me one day "I hardly even can remember what it used to be like". She no longer needed the physical expression through the arthritis because she could now articulate her emotional self much more readily. It felt as though Diana was integrating the psyche into the soma as Winnicott (1966) described.

By allowing the body in the room it does not seem to matter which aspect of their self the client initially presents to the therapist. If the therapist expects and is prepared to hold the unity of a person, their wholeness can be explored like a round sphere that can be turned over and over, allowing the different aspects to be brought into the light. In my practice those that come because of their physical symptoms will often begin with the body as a way into their other dimensions as described by Wilber (2000).

Summary

My own transformation as a MindBody psychotherapist has been, and will continue to be, a life-long process. My process continues to be about accepting, acknowledging and using the whole of my being that is available to me, to invite the whole of the other in. This means placing value on all that I think, feel, know, and have experience of; and trusting that it may be significant in the work. This means a dream needs to be valued as much as a piece of empirical research; it means understanding an aspect of quantum physics might be as enlightening as a spiritual moment of deep connection with a client; it means my embodied response to my client's embodied story needs to be felt and listened to and taken seriously as evidence of something happening in the work.

As I have shown, a MindBody philosophy is a way of being rather than a formulaic technique; it is that which allows me to extend how I already practise as a psychotherapist to be inclusive and confident in working with the body. A way of being that allows an openness to my limitations as a practitioner and works to build a framework of support to address blind spots and areas of vulnerability. This framework comprises weekly individual and group supervision, and surrounding myself with a community of complementary, like-minded MindBody practitioners. In this way I feel my practice continues to be enhanced and simultaneously challenged to address the tacit and often unconscious norms of dichotomous thinking.

References

Bakal, D. (1999). *Minding the body—clinical uses of somatic awareness*. New York: The Guilford Press.

Broom, B. (1997). *Somatic illness and the patient's other story: a practical integrative approach to disease for doctors and psychotherapists*. New York: Free Association Books.

Groddeck, G. (1977). *The meaning of illness. Selected psychoanalytic writings*. London: The Hogarth Press and The Psychoanalytic Institute.

Grosz, E. (1994). *Volatile bodies: Toward a corporeal feminism*. Bloomington: Indiana University Press.

Malick, T. (2011). *The tree of life*. Los Angeles: Foxlight Studios.
McDougall, J. (1989). *Theatres of the body. A psychoanalytic approach to psychosomatic illness*. London: Free Association Books.
Mehl-Madrona, L. (2005). Connectivity and healing: some hypotheses about the phenomenon and how to study it. *Advances, 21, (1)*: 12–28
Wilber, K. (2000). *A brief history of everything*. Boston: Shambhala.
Winnicot, D. (1953). Transitional objects and transitional phenomena—a study of the first not-me possession. *The International Journal of Psychoanalysis, 34*: 89–97.
Winnicott, D. (1966). Psycho-somatic illness in its positive and negative aspects. *The International Journal of Psychoanalysis, 47*: 510–516.

CHAPTER SIX

The gift of illness: inviting physical symptoms to guide personal growth

Renske van den Brink

The transition from working as a traditional general medical practitioner (GP) to a MindBody therapist has been a gradual process beginning with my own experience of illness. The process has been intensely personal and deeply transformative. The professional challenges entailed have led to a radical re-shaping of my work. I will share some core aspects of my own journey, and then address theoretical and clinical tensions I have had to resolve in order to feel grounded in my work.

Introduction

I began my career as a GP in a low decile community, carrying a heavy obstetrics load. I worked as a part-time clinician at the local hospice, and enjoyed the challenge of doing some extramural study. It was exciting and satisfying, but gradually the volume of work and the burden of the multiple demands on my time tipped the scales, and I became increasingly stressed and unwell. This eventually resulted in what I would now call "burn out".

Nothing I learned at medical school had prepared me for the long and frustratingly slow process ahead. I spent the next year not working, and searching for my own healing. Initially I sought help from many different health practitioners who typically asserted in a persuasive and kindly way that their approaches were certain to succeed. The navigation of my subsequent disappointment and self-blame, when I still found myself unwell after these treatments, added difficulty to difficulty. My experience of the medical model reinforced a belief that the answer was outside myself; I just had to find the right medication, the right physiotherapist, psychotherapist, or some other therapist whose particular skill or expertise would get rid of my troublesome symptoms.

For many months I struggled to avoid what I now know was the central issue for me; that my illness had a meaning. It was largely to do with me. The illusion of an external cause, and an external cure, functioned only to protect me from the painful and unpalatable truth; this illness was mostly to do with me, and the way I was living my life. I couldn't work for that year because I had to surrender to what initially felt like the collapse of my being. I had to stop helping others in order to have time for myself, and for what my body was urgently trying to communicate. I understand now that this struggle was ultimately a reflection of my gradual movement from a world underpinned by the assumptions of the dualistic medical model which I had been grounded in, to a new possibility of well-being built on a unitary model of personhood. This was the radical paradigm shift I needed in order to re-evaluate and engage with what my body was expressing

What follows is, firstly, an exploration of the theoretical underpinnings of that movement process, and, secondly, the application of these ideas to my work.

The conceptual bog

Medical school learning was grounded in the positivist paradigm, as described by the early nineteenth century philosopher Auguste Comte (see Giddings & Grant, 2002). Objectivity and systematic observation were emphasized, and hypotheses were tested through experimentation and verification. Without ever questioning this ontology, I embraced the concept that truth is only what can be discovered as an objective reality, and that scientific research methods are required to prove its validity (Giddings & Grant, 2002). My success as a medical student depended on the amount of factual information I could retrieve and regurgitate accurately. The patient was presented as a combination of signs and symptoms, which I was then required to interpret in order to make my diagnosis. The patient resembled a machine in need of repair and maintenance by the doctor (mechanic). In this model, the body is implicitly viewed as separate from the mind, and illness is divided into either real, organic disease which has an objectively measurable cause, or less real, functional, illnesses which originate in the mind (Broom, 2000). Furthermore, as an impressionable, enthusiastic young doctor, I unquestioningly took on the role of "doctor as God". This helped my professional confidence, and massaged my ego; but added a great burden of responsibility to provide my patients with all the answers and solutions.

When hospital medicine succeeded medical school in my learning process, the metaphor of the body-as-a-machine was closely matched and reinforced by the increasing dependence on technology at the doctor-patient interface (Samson, 1999). The value placed on technology as healer seemed to outweigh even my newly learned medical knowledge, let alone any interpersonal skills I may have contributed in the consultation.

When I entered general practice, however, it was the biopsychosocial model (Engel, 1977) and the patient-centred method of consultation style which became more central to my clinical practice (Boyle, Dwinnell & Platt, 2005; Hawken, 2005; Silverman, Kurtz & Draper, 1998; Stewart, M., Brown, J. B., Donner, A., McWhinney, I. R., Oates, J., Weston, W. W. & Jordan, J. 2000). During my GP training I learned to use role plays and the actor-simulated interview, which enabled me to begin to include the patient's illness experience in my diagnostic formulations. It was a relief to find others (Epstein, R. M., Shields, C. G., Meldrum, S. C., Fiscella, K., Carroll, J. & Carney, P. A., 2006, p. 806), when writing about the patient-centred consultation, stating: "… we need to understand the patient as a person, rather than as a cluster of attributes." Although the mind and body were still viewed as relatively separate, the psychosocial context was brought into the foreground, and this certainly improved my capacity for rapport with my patients.

Although in the biopsychosocial model the patient did receive an opportunity to explore their emotional experience, there was still a fundamental dualism; dividing illness into either the mental or physical domains. If I, as the GP, could not find a physical cause for their symptoms, and make significant progress to resolve it, the next step was a referral to a community mental health team in the hope that a psychiatrist would address the assumed and yet ill-defined psychological issues. Frequently, such mental health teams, equally grounded in psychiatric versions of the dualistic model, were unable to make a difference either.

As the GP, I would be left with a sense of failure; I could not help my patient effectively and they in turn, seemed stuck. The patients were often equally disempowered. They experienced themselves as increasingly pathologised, resulting in self-blame, lowered self-esteem, and, often, unnecessarily reliant on antidepressants, powerful analgesics and tranquilizers.

Thus, dominated by this traditional reductionist biomedical model based in a dualistic paradigm, the healthcare system is left to struggle with unresolved symptomatology, increasing patient dependency, and unnecessary health spending, as it attempts to address the wrong problem. A different model and a different kind of clinical exploration are needed for these people and their doctors.

Learning to listen

My own experience of illness took me on a deep personal journey of exploration of how issues in our lives are represented in our body. I entered a process of explorative psychotherapy for myself, and began to connect with my own story and grapple with the existential questions of "Who am I?" In particular, I was facing the challenge of "Who am I if I can't work? Who am I if I can't help others? Who am I if I need help myself?"

Intrigued by the inner workings of the psyche, I enrolled in a Diploma of Psychosynthesis Counselling, setting me on a path of developing my own private practice as a counsellor, whilst still working part-time as a GP. This was a very humbling time. I had a great deal of "un-learning" to do. I had to set aside my prescriptive and outcome-focussed style of being with patients. I gradually learned to inhibit my tendency to give lots of good advice and, instead, listen actively as deeply as possible to where the patient was at.

Learning how to listen is not a high priority in medicine. The great majority of time at medical school is spent learning how the body works, how it goes wrong, and how to fix it. All of that is important, but, sadly, the patient's story is typically not allowed or is cut short soon after we hear which body part is "going wrong". Once the doctor has become mentally oriented to the body system in which the troublesome symptom belongs, a focussed functional enquiry begins. For example, a patient with chest pain triggers a cardiovascular review, a stomach pain points to the gastrointestinal system, and bladder discomfort requires a urinary system review. Of course that is not all that doctors are supposed to do, and I did learn to ask, "Who lives at home and what do you do for a job?" However, by then I had usually already decided what the diagnosis was, and often I had the prescription completed in my mind, if not already written. It was too late to really listen to the patient's illness experience, or, even more importantly, to the story of what was going on in their lives when their symptoms began.

The time constraint inherent in a busy primary care setting is often seen by doctors as a barrier to deepening a patient's story, and certainly I felt this frustration. However, it is possible for health practitioners to use the time that they have with patients in a more "story-centred" way, and I began to explore how to maximise patient contact time, without necessarily needing to extend it (Dugdale, Epstein & Pantilat, 1999). This led eventually into teaching communication skills to doctors and health professionals, using professional actors and role plays. Experience revealed that it is not how much time we have that is the limiting factor; it is how we use the time. I have developed a structure for the consultation called the Wine Glass Model (see diagram below) which has helped many health professionals to inhibit their natural tendencies to narrow the focus early on in the consultation with medicalized closed questions; and instead allow the patient to take the stage first, with a spacious invitation to tell the story of their illness experience.

The 'Wineglass model'

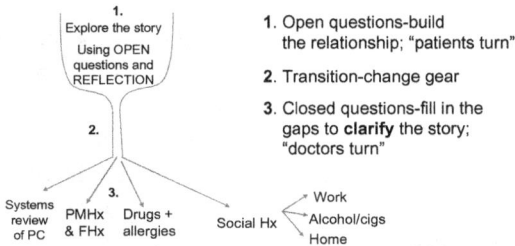

1. Explore the story
Using OPEN questions and REFLECTION

2.

3.
Systems review of PC   PMHx & FHx   Drugs + allergies   Social Hx   Work   Alcohol/cigs   Home

1. Open questions-build the relationship; "patients turn"

2. Transition-change gear

3. Closed questions-fill in the gaps to clarify the story; "doctors turn"

www.connectcomm.co.nz

An example is that, assuming the doctor has six minutes to take a history, they use the first three to four minutes to ask open questions and reflect the concerns of the patient. Rapport then builds quickly, and that is also the time to ask a question such as "what was happening at the time the symptom started?" Then the last two minutes can be used to rapidly fill in the gaps with closed questions such as "have you had a fever, or does the pain radiate anywhere?"

When the patient's illness experience is valued in the medical consultation, improved outcomes are seen on many levels (Boyle, D., Dwinnell, B. & Platt, F., 2005; Hawken, 2005; Silverman, J., Kurtz, S. & Draper, J., 1998). I have found that there is a profound wisdom in the symptom itself. It is not just something to be removed. It becomes highly functional to pay attention to the story behind the symptom (Broom, 2000; Chiozza, 1999; Groddeck, 1977; McDougall, 1989). If we can suspend the need to solve the problem for the first few minutes, we may be able to learn what it is that is being expressed by the body. This requires the practitioner to put together the possible links between the story of the symptom, and the symptom itself. We create the space for the symptom to communicate meaning.

In mainstream general practice, however, many patients come with the familiar dualistic reductionist model inherent in their strong conviction that the doctor is being paid to fix their problem. This is particularly problematic when the presenting issue is something like chronic pain, relentless fatigue, or a frenetically busy corporate business person who complains of frequent illnesses such as colds and viral infections. These conditions are seldom simple to solve or quick to respond to conventional treatment. A dramatic shift is required of the practitioner to resist moving quickly into problem-solving; and instead listen and explore what is going on with the patient. The spoken or unspoken demand to fix the patient is difficult for most practitioners, and particularly for doctors, because it projects onto the clinician the belief that the answer is both outside the patient and up to the clinician to find. As doctors we are easy repositories for such projections. Terms like gold standard and evidence-based practice reinforce an almost fundamentalist conviction that we are first and foremost right. Although protocols and guidelines clearly have inherent value, the shadow side of these terms is that they give both the practitioner and the patient a false sense of certainty, and cause foreclosure on the patient's story. How can we be open to allow meaning to be revealed by a patient's story when we have already jumped to a conclusion concerning what the problem is and what is needed? An invaluable aid for this dramatic shift is to prioritize diagnostic self-control. This is comparable to delayed gratification, and requires the doctor to delay their diagnosis and listen to the patient's story first. I wait and explore and truly listen with all of my being to what the patient is communicating to me. This means listening with more than my ears.

I watch, feel, notice my own physical and emotional responses and tune in energetically to get as close as possible to what is emerging. This means prioritising my own receptivity over my capacity to give a solution and creates an environment whereby the patient is invited to reveal more of who they really are. They are free to tell their story and be seen as a fully unique and diverse human being, rather than a poor collection of symptoms.

Empathy extended

In the patient-centred model we are asked to put ourselves in the patient's shoes, and I have spent many hours teaching this concept to health professionals. I remind them that empathy is easy when we like the patient and they are similar to us. The challenge is to remain empathic when the patient is different to us; they have different values, different politics, or they may be someone we disapprove of. We are still required to be non-judgmental and remain able to empathize and understand. However, in my learning as a counsellor and a budding psychotherapist, I have been challenged to take the concept of empathy one step further. Donna Orange suggests that "if I want to understand I must go toward the utterer, not force the utterer to come to me" (2011, p. 5). That is, to abandon my idea of the patient, and allow their world to be mine. Personally, I have found this to be profoundly unsettling. I have to be willing to let go of my familiar territory, the known world of hypothesis and diagnosis. Instead, to surrender to the chaos of the patient's immediate lived experience; allowing it to affect me and to influence me in the direction of where we go together.

As I began to develop confidence in working in a more holistic way, it became important to be around like-minded people because I still felt I had one foot in each camp: on the one hand the reductive biomedical camp and on the other the MindBody or whole person care camp. The New Zealand MindBody Trust was formed in 2004, creating a unique community for the expression of integrated ways of working with health issues. My ongoing search for a new body of knowledge that would bring together my skills as both a counsellor and a doctor, finally took me to study at AUT University in the Post Graduate Diploma of MindBody Healthcare. This was a very spacious and grounded forum in which to explore in detail the many layers and dimensions of what was emerging for me.

A new paradigm

In this stimulating environment of postgraduate learning, I was well-resourced to develop a new and sound theoretical framework to hold what had previously been a predominantly instinctive drive towards prioritising the patient's story. Many philosophical questions arose, demanding ontological and epistemological insights, and revealing theories of knowledge and truth I had not previously considered. How do we know the things we know? And what is the reference point for that which we unquestioningly know as truth?

Qualitative research theories offered an expansive structure with which to underpin my new experience and ideas. I learned that the interpretive paradigm contrasts sharply with the positivist position, in its desire to "understand what it is to be human and what meaning people attach to the events in their lives" (Giddings & Grant, 2002 p. 16). From a philosophical point of view it was first Heidegger (1962), and later Merleau-Ponty (1962), who argued that the fundamental biological unit of information is not merely true or false, but is rather a rich interconnected unit of form and meaning, a sensory gestalt represented in language as story (Griffith & Elliot Griffith, 1994).

Combined with this philosophical paradigm shift I was fascinated to discover the flood of new research that has been published over the last 20 years which supports the physiological links between stressful life events and physical health (Irwin, 2008; Tosevski & Milovancevic, 2006). Vaccine studies show that in people looking after a relative with dementia, stress results in a weaker antibody and virus specific T-cell response. Similarly progression from HIV to AIDS was two to three times higher in men who were above the median level for stress. Wound healing was also shown to be twenty-four to forty per cent slower in patients suffering above median levels of stress. These studies represent a small number of an increasingly strong body of work that demonstrates a clear link between stress and the quality of body function (Glaser & Kiecolt-Glaser, 2009).

A new way of practicing

As I began to shift into longer appointments and deeper work with patients, I found my private practice as a counsellor and MindBody therapist was growing, so over time, I gradually let go of the more traditional GP work. I learned to value my own bodily responses to differing work environments and I found that my own usual stress-related symptoms settled down, leaving me feeling more energized and congruent in myself. It was a difficult decision to leave traditional general practice, but gradually I realized that the tensions came from the pressure to produce traditional outcomes within a limited time-frame. First, fifteen and then twenty minute consultations were not long enough, and I realized that my tendency to explore and deepen was creating a dilemma in itself. It seemed that I needed a more spacious structure in order to do more of what I was good at. So I moved to working with longer appointments and ongoing sessions with fewer patients. I still reference myself as a GP, in that I work with primary healthcare issues, but now I use a more spacious psychotherapeutic frame in which to help those same patients.

As a counsellor who is also a GP, my medical experience and knowledge combine with my therapist skills to support working in a holistic way with complex and challenging clinical scenarios. I increasingly notice that the disconnection between a person's inner experience and the way that they present themselves to the world seems to result in the generation of chronic tension which can then manifest somewhere in the body. It is as though there is an inner versus outer differential, which requires an exhausting amount of energy to manage, and results in physical distress. The body receives two conflicting directives creating a bind and often an unspeakable dilemma. An example is a person who experiences an inner impulse to "mobilize for anger" in order to express themselves, but is then inhibited by a habitual silencing of the self in order to fit in with social norms.

The MindBody connection

Judy was a high achieving business woman in her early thirties who presented with symptoms of debilitating fatigue and low mood. She came from a family that valued achievement and had high expectations, but provided little love and support to meet the demands that were set. She avoided conflict, fearing disapproval, and her self-esteem was closely tied to her achievements. These appeared to be the predisposing factors (Mayou & Farmer, 2002) to getting unwell. Her fatigue began after her partner pressured her to take six months off work for an overseas trip at a vital time in her career when she felt she needed to remain at work or lose her position in the company. This was the precipitating event. She felt unable to refuse him, and also unable to negotiate time off work because her seniority in the company had rapidly progressed. This internal conflict became too much to bear, and when she fell ill with a viral infection her recovery was delayed, and she began to experience increasing fatigue. She describes: "I feel like I'm spending every non-working hour in bed …. I can hardly drag myself out of there to go to work, it's all too much effort." This culminated in having to take extended time off work.

There were other factors which perpetuated her symptoms, including having few friends who really understood her. They tended to off-load onto her. She felt compelled to put her own needs aside, and help others even when it wasn't her responsibility. Judy felt increasingly isolated, guilty, and under pressure.

Her recovery entailed making space for the part of herself she called Tired Judy; a part that didn't want to go overseas with her partner and felt angry that he would not consider her needs, but also scared about standing up for herself in case he left her. Creating a safe non-judgmental and supportive space for Tired Judy enabled her to gain confidence and find the words to express how she felt verbally rather than having her body act it out physically. Gradually she began to feel more congruent as her internal experience was more accurately reflected in how she presented herself to her colleagues, family and friends. She had to learn how to say "no", how to stay connected to someone with whom she disagreed, and how to bear the tension of feeling disapproved of; all without losing faith in herself.

Intimate confrontation

Many of us know the relieving experience of being able to blame someone else for our distress, in stark contrast to the pain of having to admit our own part in something that has gone wrong. In a related way, we see the process of a patient perceiving the symptom as representive of a connection between subjective and physical dimensions, and then coming to an acceptance that it is their own personal issue that needs solving; this pathway is central to healing. However, this process can be very personally challenging and requires courage, trust and safety. So the practitioner is required to be non-judgmental, empathic and genuinely willing to get alongside the patient in order to create a safe non-blaming space in which to explore the meaning of the symptom.

In my experience, the more serious the patient's physical symptom, the more radical the response that is required of the patient, and perhaps even the more empathic the practitioner needs to be. A person who is in strong denial, in need of protection from what is too painful to bear, needs to feel safe and understood to entertain the possibility that their inner difficulties are in fact directly affecting their physical experience. When we as practitioners challenge patients or give them feedback that is hard for them to hear and accept, we need to be able to trade on the strength of the therapeutic bond. When the empathic connection is strong, and the rapport reliably robust, the relationship can stand the test.

Melinda is forty two years old, and was referred by her GP with a two year history of sleep disturbance, nightmares and fertility issues. Several times a week she would scream loudly in her sleep, and then wake up in terror. The fertility issues were complex and multi-layered, causing a lot of distress for her and her partner of ten years. She was initially very reluctant to come for therapy, presenting as warm and polite, but strongly denying that there was anything wrong emotionally. In particular, she was very reluctant to explore any possibility there might be a connection between a sexual trauma event, that happened when she was seventeen, and the fact that her nightmares began after a termination of pregnancy which occurred two years ago. Initially I was not sure either about what the connection actually was, but it seemed important to hold the two events side by side until things became clearer.

Very early in our work, I was strongly aware of a tension between her impatience to get rid of the nightmares, and a reluctance to allow her early story to matter at all. In the beginning she just could not bear it when I brought the threads together. She became very distressed, at times "going blank" (dissociating) when asked direct questions about what she was experiencing. This in itself was a strong clue that the topic I was raising had a deeper meaning for her. I also sensed how brittle our therapeutic alliance was as I gingerly walked the line between upsetting her by drawing attention to what I saw, and building the relationship with acceptance, empathy and compassion.

Brian Broom (1997, and personal communication) discusses clinical intimacy, and what he calls "intimate confrontation", that right mixture of delicate empathy and goodwill towards the patient, matched by a determination not to be distracted from the underlying truths behind the physical manifestation. There must be a willingness to endure the discomfort for both the patient and the therapist as they get close to the intolerable place. The practitioner has to get this balance right; too much confrontation and the client disengages as the threat is too much to handle, and too little challenge results in getting nowhere and progress being delayed. Resistance is "a way of coping" or protection; an armouring that defends against something that is too much to bear, and that has a very important function for the client (Soth, 1999). We need to ask without judgment: "What is being defended against? What about this is too hard to bear?"

Even when a patient is not ready to explore their emotional experience, and wants the practitioner to take responsibility for the healing process, rather than labelling them as resistant or difficult, we have the opportunity to include the resistance as part of the meaning making, to allow it to be valued as having an important role in the genesis of the whole story. The resistance can thus be viewed as a symptom in just the same way that the nightmare or the infertility is a symptom. Both can be seen as symbols of an internal process requiring trust and safety to be established before the meaning of the symbol can be revealed and understood by both the client and the practitioner. Additionally, the practitioner needs to be willing to hold their own interpretations, and first attend to what the client needs in order to move towards the potentially frightening truth of the meaning of the symptom. Sometimes clients need time to build trust in the therapeutic relationship, sometimes they need time to build their own self-esteem, sometimes the practitioner just needs to engage with humility and patience as the process unfolds, perhaps in a direction that is not at all what was expected.

> After about eight sessions Melinda tentatively ventured into exploring her story of the rape she experienced at age seventeen. As she began describing her somatic experience during the rape, she raised her arms as if to ward off the perpetrator, which suddenly resonated with a pivotal aspect in her nightmares in which she always woke up with her arms raised in front of her face, combined with a feeling of profound terror and the vision of a

menacing shadowy face. This was very shocking for her as she realised within herself that the nightmare and the rape were indeed
intimately connected. However, by now, her increased inner resilience, combined with her growing trust in me gave her the confidence to allow these difficult threads to be brought together and
she was able to begin the work of processing her trauma story.

Since this time her nightmares have changed, initially becoming less violent, and now less frequent. To begin with they were
occurring several times a week, now once a month, if at all. In fact,
Melinda is now able to respond to the nightmares as a message
that requires attention to her inner world. She is also beginning to
understand that the termination of pregnancy, which triggered the
nightmares, holds deep shame and sadness for her, and is now very
connected with her current difficulty in falling pregnant again.
Accepting the meaning of her symptoms is a slow and sad process for Melinda. The cost for her has been to give up the protective
belief that all the troubling parts of her story have no relevance
to her current emotional pain. It has resulted in an excruciatingly
painful process as she allows herself to begin the grieving of all
that she has lost as a woman, and all that she never had as a daughter. What she has gained however, is a deep connection with her
authentic self and this is steadily transmitting itself to her partner
as their intimacy and mutuality grows through the process.

Confrontation is in many instances an inevitable part of working with
physical illness in a MindBody way, because it implicitly and explicitly
challenges the common understanding of illness. The idea that meaning
and physicality belong in the same space is radical in our contemporary
technological and compartmentalized world. Even the biopsychosocial model of disease still keeps physical and mental aspects separate.
Patients come to doctors expecting a physical answer, and it is confronting to discover there are clinicians who believe and practise otherwise.
Yet it is a wise and ancient concept that there is no separateness between
mind and body, that everything is connected and interdependent.
Traditions as old as Indian Ayurveda and Traditional Chinese Medicine
maintain that there is no separation between mind and body, or body
and spirit; or whatever other aspects of being we might use to describe
what it is to be human. Broom (2003) takes this a step further when he
explores the implications of interconnectedness of meaning and physical illness, and how the body can hold a specific symbolism which fits

with the patient's story. He calls this phenomenon "somatic metaphor" or "symbolic illness" and outlines how listening to the language which our patients use can be just as revealing as using our more usual diagnostic tools. Listening more deeply involves listening for these symbols and metaphors whilst the patient describes their experience, and in particular, their symptoms.

The symbolic symptom

I am currently working with Simon, an intelligent, articulate fifty year old man who initially presented with rapid onset of rheumatoid arthritis, work and family stress combining to the point where he felt he had little control over his life. He had to take six months off from the most meaningful part of his work, and he was unable to walk around the block due to pain in his knees and feet. Simon had always had difficulty expressing anger, and over the years he had learned to internalise negative experiences, presenting himself as flexible, easily pleased, and quick to forgive. However, tension in his family of origin was gradually rising and becoming harder to bear. Underneath his easy-going and cheerful persona, he was angry and frustrated. It was as though his rheumatoid symptoms of pain and stiffness were saying: "actually being so flexible is not working for me; what about me and my needs?" Simon gradually became used to the process of weekly therapy and more comfortable with making space for his deeper and more difficult feelings. He began to articulate and express his rage, which was a totally new experience for him. As he gave himself full permission to be furious with his brother, I asked him how it felt to be so strongly in his anger. "Like a shot of Prednisone!" he answered immediately. As he heard himself say that, he realised that owning and expressing his anger was as therapeutic as taking his rheumatoid medicines. Letting go of his anger was relieving in that his inner tension lessened as his anger was fervently expressed in a safe place.

At this time, Simon also became much more confident in letting his doctors know more of what was not going well for him and this resulted in a change of medication, which, combined with his work on his emotional issues, has resulted in him coming off Prednisone altogether. He has found particular value in the concept of congruence, whereby he aims to harmonize his inner and outer experience by being more transparent in his relationships. This includes saying the difficult things that may risk disapproval, or make others consider him less flexible, rather than the alternative which requires him to manage the steep differential of inner struggle with outer tranquillity. Simon has had a radical improvement of his symptoms, no longer relying on a walking stick and managing to exercise relatively comfortably as long as he stays connected to his needs.

Listening for the quality of the presenting symptom adds another dimension to the information that is already there in the story.

This became apparent in my work with Dave who presented with sudden onset of anaphylaxis involving swelling of his lips and tongue with accompanying chest tightness and bronchoconstriction. He was fully investigated at the Immunology Clinic and was found not to be allergic to any food or environmental allergens. However, his symptoms began in the context of a chronically difficult relationship with his partner of six years, which became suddenly much worse following the birth of Dave's first grandson. His partner had always been very jealous and controlling, and now she had a strongly negative reaction to Dave's enthusiasm as a grandfather. This resulted in an acute escalation of his own internal tension which became unbearable for him, because he had no words for how to express his dissatisfaction with her verbally. The swelling of the tongue seemed to represent a paralysis of his capacity to speak out for himself. He was extremely fearful of her response to him, a fear embedded in his role as the peacekeeper in the relationship. His anaphylaxis required emergency treatment and transfer to hospital several times and when we debriefed this together we realised that the symptom was saying "This is an emergency, it's a matter of life and death." It was as though his anaphylaxis was telling him that he was at a crisis point in his life; he could not go on in this soul-destroying relationship. His own words were, "It would be the death of me!" Attending to this knowledge has required Dave to make radical and urgent changes in order to preserve his right to live in a congruent and authentic way. As a result of this knowledge, and his increasing confidence in saying what he needs to his partner, his anaphylaxis symptoms have disappeared, other than a warning tingling in his mouth which occurs if there is something difficult that needs to be said. Things are not yet settled for him, and he continues to struggle with finding a strong authentic place for himself, but he has gained a newfound confidence that he can trust his body to give him feedback with his experience in relationships.

Conclusion

In these few examples it becomes clear that illness is not a random event, not just something to be got rid of as soon as possible. The profound wisdom inherent in the symptom becomes a gift when we can spaciously respond to what is needed to find balance and wholeness.

Finding the connection between symptom and meaning has been central to the healing process in these examples, and it is tempting to extrapolate this to all health scenarios. However, there is a danger of imposing meaning onto all physical symptoms in a way which can then become as fundamentalist and fixed as the dualistic medical model itself. Illness is most often multi-factorial. The advantage of including meaning is that this is the one part of the puzzle we can at least do something about, and most often the personal learning is transferable to many life situations in a beneficial way.

The MindBody practitioner requires an alert and flexible approach which can include matter and spirit, body and mind. The Japanese concept of *Shosin* (beginner's mind) invites us to have the attitude of openness, eagerness and lack of preconceptions in our most expert moments. This requires a deep humility on the part of the practitioner, and I believe that when this attitude is combined simultaneously with a paradoxical attentiveness to having a rigorous theoretical MindBody framework, an optimum healing space can freely emerge.

The history of healing on our planet reveals vastly diverse world views, ranging from shamanism to ancient mystical traditions underpinning Indian Ayurveda and traditional Chinese medicine, to the intellectualized modern Western Cartesian dualism giving rise to modernist biomedicine and its highly technological emphasis. A modern holistic MindBody approach calls forth a capacity to utilize not only the comfortable world of cognitive and technical knowledge, but also to yield to the unfamiliar mysterious and disturbing world of myself, the Other, and the related complex intersubjective fields. In so doing, we can then use the ancient lens of balance and interconnectedness to focus our sophisticated modern medical knowledge.

References

Broom, B. (1997). *Somatic illness and the patient's other story*. London: Free Association Books.

Broom, B. (2000). Medicine and story: A novel clinical panorama arising from a unitary mind/body approach to physical illness. *Advances in Mind-Body Medicine, 16*: 161–207.

Broom, B. (2003). Somatic metaphor: A clinical phenomenon pointing to a new model of disease, personhood, and physical reality. *Advances in Mind-Body Medicine, 18(1)*: 17–29.

Boyle, D., Dwinnell, B. & Platt, F. (2005). Invite, listen and summarise: A patient-centred communication technique. *Academic Medicine, 80*: 29–32.

Chiozza, L. A. (1999). *Why do we fall ill?* Madison, CT: Psychosocial Press.

Dugdale, D. C., Epstein, R. & Pantilat, S. Z. (1999). Time and the patient-physician relationship. *Journal of General Internal Medicine, 14*: S34-S40.

Engel, G. L. (1977). The need for a new medical model: A challenge for bio-medicine. *Science, 196*: 129–36.

Epstein, R. M., Shields, C. G., Meldrum, S. C., Fiscella, K., Carroll, J. & Carney, P. A (2006). Physicians' responses to patients' medically unex-plained symptoms. *Psychosomatic Medicine, 68(2)*, 269–276.

Giddings, L. S. & Grant, B. (2002). Making sense of methodologies: A paradigm framework for the novice researcher. *Contemporary Nurse, 13(1)*: 10–27.

Glaser, R. & Kiecolt-Glaser, J. (2009). Stress damages immune system and health. *Discovery medicine, 5(26)*: 165–169.

Griffith, J. L. & Elliot Griffith, M. (1994). *The body speaks: Therapeutic dialogues for mind-body problems*. New York: Basic Books.

Groddeck, G. (1977). *The meaning of illness*. New York: International Universities Press.

Gunton, C. E. (1993). *The one, the three and the many: God, creation, and the culture of modernity*. Cambridge, UK: Cambridge University Press.

Hawken, S. J. (2005). Good communication skills: Benefits for doctors and patients. *New Zealand Family Physician, 32(3)*: 185–189.

Heidegger, M. (1962). *Being and time*. Oxford, UK: Blackwell Publishing.
Irwin, M. R. (2008). Human Psychoneuroimmunology: 20 Years of discovery. *Brain, Behaviour and Immunity, 22: 129–139*.
Mayou, R. & Farmer, A. (2002). Functional somatic symptoms and syndromes. *British Medical Journal 325*: 265.
McDougall, J. (1989). *Theatres of the body: A psychoanalytic approach to illness*. New York: W. W. Norton.
Merleau-Ponty, M. (1962). *The phenomenology of perception*. London: Routledge.
Orange, D. (2011). *The suffering stranger: Hermeneutics for everyday clinical practice*. London: Routledge.
Samson, C. (1999). Biomedicine and the body. In C. Samson (Ed.), *Health Studies: A critical and cross-cultural reader* (pp. 3–21).
Silverman, J., Kurtz, S. & Draper, J. (1998.) *Skills for communicating with patients*. Oxon: Radcliffe Medical Press.
Soth, M (1999). Relating to and with the objectified body. *Self and Society 27(1)*: 32–38.
Stewart, M., Brown, J. B., Donner, A., McWhinney, I. R., Oates, J., Weston, W. W. & Jordan, J. (2000). The impact of patient-centred care on outcomes. *The Journal of Family Practice, 49(9)*: 796–804.
Tosevski, D. & Milovancevic, M. (2006). Stress and physical health. *Current Opinion in Psychiatry, 19(2)*: 184–190.

CHAPTER SEVEN

Professional earthquake and aftershocks

Karen Lindsay

The tectonic plates underpinning my personal life and clinical practice have shifted, and keep shifting. This began in 2009 when, as a rheumatology specialist, I migrated to New Zealand and took temporary work in the Immunology department at Auckland City Hospital. I received much more than I bargained for. I found myself working alongside an immunologist who was also a psychotherapist, and a MindBody physician, and suddenly the ground underneath me was moving. My paradigms, the foundations of my thinking, were being challenged and changed.

I will give an account of my experience of becoming a MindBody clinician in the hospital system, but, reader be warned, this may engender a sense of frustration, incompleteness, and not knowing. I hope I might be forgiven this. The task I have taken on is gargantuan. When the hospital system has changed to incorporate MindBody perspectives for the benefit of patients I will feel that I am there. This is a long way off.

I discovered that the term MindBody is commonly used by a network of New Zealand clinicians, and reflects the recognized difficulties of thinking about the mind and body as one entity, both dimensions constituting whole human beings (Broom, 2007). The MindBody approach sets out to overcome this dualism in healthcare, this split between the mind and body that penetrates our language, our thinking, our research, and its funding; and the care provided by our public and private health services. Whilst I was aware there were limitations to what medicine could achieve, I was not aware this philosophical foundation was called dualism, and would not have been able to articulate it as a problem, let alone question it. However this has all shifted. Change has been sudden, and the learning curve has been steep, and at times disturbing. The entire experience has been transformative. What is remarkable is that I have begun to see consistent and compelling relationships between unique psychosocial stressors and all types of inflammatory diseases. I never saw them before. Others certainly have (Broom, 2007; Brook, 1994; Hoyt, 1957; Groddeck, 1932), but it is not part of physician training either here or in the United Kingdom.

I joined a post-graduate university programme in MindBody Healthcare. Formal study of the theoretical concepts behind this approach has taken me to non-biomedical literature and to psychotherapy in particular, but also to knowledge from many other disciplines such as neuroscience, sociology, anthropology and ethics. Working alongside Dr Broom, I have been able to think about and discuss patients in a non-dualistic way case by case. I now grapple with utilizing the approach in rheumatology and inflammatory eye clinics, and I think I may be one of the only people to try and do so. I feel like a pioneer and an outsider.

Working in the Immunology clinics and seeing how stories shed light on the occurrence of disease was what first disrupted my dualistic thinking. For example, chronic urticaria is a debilitating condition where people get itchy red hives on their skin. Antihistamines, and sometimes steroids, are needed to suppress it. With the MindBody approach, such patients often do remarkably well compared with those on medication. But it contradicts the way I have been trained to see disease as independent from the person, and to be tackled with medications. Despite this, I have now seen numerous examples where there has been a consistent and congruent story behind the triggering and maintenance of the particular disorder. This experience has allowed me to see beyond the symptoms, to the embodied nature of stress and story, and to learn the novelty and value of using this approach, as well as to see how difficult it is to challenge dualism in clinical practice.

Frequently, the hospital system and the patients appear to collude in keeping the mind and body separate. The MindBody approach, essentially, confronts that problem. It means that I have to listen to the unique story of the individual, to get at the emotional undercurrent of what has happened to them, and then attempt to frame the symptoms as uniquely meaningful in order that they might be able to change their way of being in relation to themselves and others. The challenge for me now is how to engage the patient and steer them against the tendency to look outward for a cause, guiding them to look inward for answers. The template for this process is no longer merely the diagnosis, but a felt sense of being with a person and their story. A totally different landscape is visible if the patient is willing to work with it. I am now doing this with every patient that I see.

> One patient had severe recurrent urticaria, and required several different antihistamines. The patient said the problem started after a phone argument with his new employer while he was on holiday. While many workers were put off by this employer's angry and superior attitude, my patient chose to work with him. They spent weekends and nights away together on projects outside town. Although he found this person unbearable, the situation continued for three years. He said he stayed because the money was very good even though his quality of life was deteriorating. It is possible that his urticaria was totally unrelated to this story, and this would be the biomedical standpoint. It could be simply due to stress, a concept of biomechanical loading. But it could be symbolic of the anger which he had suppressed in order to tolerate the situation.
>
> I reviewed his case at group supervision meetings, and there was a period of reflection with psychotherapy colleagues before going back to the patient with a different approach. We reframed his symptoms as meaningful and related to the work situation. Since then he has gone into business with someone else, the symptoms have gone and he no longer needs medication.

Using the person-centred MindBody approach I am engaging my patients in this type of reflection. Seeing symptoms as meaningful allows patients to take decisions that are both within their power and in the interests of their health. To put this into language, I have had to resort to ideas about stress, feelings, and behaviours in relationships that need to be changed. Promoting the idea that people might get better without medication, is a very different spin for a physician.

These changes have required a personal and professional transformation. Most patients do not expect to be asked about the meaningful life experiences that may have contributed to their illnesses. They are often surprised to find that, as a specialist physician, I think that life experiences may be important. Sometimes I see what the patients cannot yet see about how their experiences appear to have affected them. All manner of unspoken resistances, or defences against seeing or feeling the impact of some experience, can be in place. Believing that the patient has the innate capacity to heal themselves is important here (Griffiths, 1994) and persisting with this approach can be difficult, because it can be very confronting for people.

Being a beginner in Immunology certainly was helpful. In some ways training and knowledge get in the way of seeing and hearing what is before us. The Buddhists advocate having "a beginners mind" and being in a new speciality enabled me to adopt this attitude. I have begun to hone my skills in uncovering meaningful stories without my specialist expertise getting in the way. In addition, I have begun to transfer the MindBody approach to rheumatology, where because of greater knowledge and training, my paradigm and worldview is less flexible. This said, taking a MindBody approach in patients with more serious and life threatening diseases has been difficult.

> A patient with psoriatic arthritis who was experiencing a flare up had been referred back to the rheumatology clinic after a period of being lost to follow up. He related that when he was a child his father often physically beat him. On one occasion, after he had told his father he had been bullied, he had slammed him against the wall, saying he had a "yellow streak down his back". The patient is in a relationship with someone his family disapprove of, and they were telling embarrassing and shameful lies about him in his close knit community.

The stress I perceived underlying his flare-up is an illustration of the congruence between the patient's subjective and medical objective realities, which can become visible in clinic. This man may need a psychotherapist to help him with his experiences from childhood. I am not a psychotherapist; however I do endeavour to hold life experiences like this as important clinical data to be taken into account. Psoriasis is a shameful and stigmatizing disease, and the current view in the biomedical literature (Jankovic, Raznatovic, Marinkovic, Maksimovic, Jankovic, & Djikanovic, 2009) is that this shame is merely due to the person's appearance, a side-effect of the condition. The MindBody approach would take the patient's shame and his psoriasis as being co-emergent dimensions, and a reflection of his life experience. Such experiences might be modified through a therapeutic relationship aimed at making conscious the link between them and his condition.

> The patient willingly told me his story, and I introduced the idea that his life experience might be meaningful in relation to his psoriasis, and also recommended treatment of his arthritis with methotrexate. He refused methotrexate because he wanted to father another child, and so we chose another drug, which he did accept. His psoriasis is still very active, and, in short, I am unable to engage this man in either a satisfactory biomedical or MindBody approach. He cannot afford a psychotherapist. I can see how his condition may have symbolic meaning for him but I cannot pursue it. However, an opportunity may arise over the coming months, and it may be that he will accept one or other of these approaches, ideally both.

I see many patients with inflammatory disease over long periods of time, and opportunities do arise to discuss openly what the underlying experiences were behind them becoming ill. Much of it is beyond my (practitioner) control. Some patients become ready in response to unseen influences in their lives. I am impressed with how patients can return having picked up on my advice, even after months of denial and resistance. I think the truth of the situation can be too hard to bear, and yet shifts may happen at any time. It appears that transformation may occur more by luck than by design.

Where did all this leave me? Three years ago I was an expert physician in rheumatology, but now I felt back to square one in terms of expertise with most patients, and, worse, without the psychotherapy skills to match. Experiencing distressing emotions in patients, and becoming aware of powerful transference and counter-transference reactions with patients I am trying to manage, is a challenge when you do not have either training or ability in this area. Some patients will be very resistant to exploring previous experiences or emotions, and some skill is needed in knowing when to pursue this in the interests of the patient. Many patients already know their experience has created or contributed to the onset or flare up in disease, but at the same time they may not know how to move on. Previously emotions were quite difficult for me to feel, and easy to avoid, but these emotions can be the pathway to healing (Broom, 2007). I now see that healing can only be fostered by attentiveness to both my own and my patients' emotional responses, allowing them to tell their story, to be as they are, and to enter into a dialogue with the patient who is finally the expert in his or her own experience. Robin Youngson's book, *Time to care*, has described wonderfully why it is mutually beneficial for us to be both more present with our patients, and to care for ourselves, and contains many pearls of wisdom which epitomize the MindBody approach (Youngson, 2012).

In the face of difficult or traumatic life experiences people are capable of many different creative solutions. I never underestimate the healing power of art, music or spiritual practice, and in fact helping patients to help themselves is the primary way in which many person-centred therapists work (Thorne, 2007). Anything that enables patients to express themselves, to use their own creative energies and imagination to integrate their emotions, experiences and stories is potentially a route to healing (McNiff, 2004). When I become attuned to what would previously be regarded as background noise in a patient's presentation, I can start to see or imagine multi-dimensional healing processes and events facilitating recovery and healing.

> Frances, a sixty-five year old woman who had symptoms of a possible lymphoma, was under investigation due to a three month history of weight loss and night sweats. Six months later, after a month long holiday in Italy, a change in diet and outlook and a new hobby of painting and walking outdoors, she returned for her follow up appointment. She was completely well and asymptomatic. Further delving showed she had been caring for her elderly mother, who was at the end of her life, when she herself got ill. When her mother died she had a renaissance of her own, and simultaneously her symptoms resolved. The investigations I requested in the meantime did not show any evidence of disease. She thought it was because she had given up coffee.

This example highlighted for me the way patients can often spontaneously do what they need to recover their wellbeing, following an inner knowledge or by using medical or alternative models, sometimes never realising the complex and multi-dimensional nature of their shifts between health and illness.

Psychodynamically-loaded clinical encounters with patients with physical disease have the potential to be harmful or healing (Stadter, 1996). I now have my own dossier of astonishing clinical experiences, of seeing stressors and stories behind real physical disease (Broom, 2007). I am being continuously taught about the MindBody connections by every patient that I see. Sometimes my only role is to hold on to both the subjective and objective dimensions of the patient, so that a kind of self-healing can occur. Medicine partitions these dimensions. At first I had to consciously fight to overcome this partitioning so that I could begin to see people as a whole again. I have found myself battling to stay afloat whilst trying to integrate my new insights into my old restricted role, which often conflicts with the biomedical efficiency required in working as a hospital consultant.

The transformation I was undergoing demanded a totally different set of skills, which may have been present in the past, but were not valued in the role of a contemporary rheumatologist. In fact, the role of the physician fosters detachment from emotions, which now needed rectifying. Skills like listening, trying to stay authentic in difficult and awkward situations, and being compassionate, instead of resorting to the mask of professionalism, did not fall under my usual banner, and were not emphasized in my training. These skills are perhaps more typical of a psychotherapist, counsellor, or nurse.

There are times when the experience of seeing the whole picture can be overwhelming and very de-stabilizing. My world becomes incoherent, and it is easier to let go and resort to dualism again. Seeing meaningful disease everywhere, even beyond the clinic, such as in my personal life and history, which I had never previously considered, is actually frightening. I find it hard to believe the healthcare system can ignore it so consistently. My desire to help remains, but the change required can feel too great, beyond my abilities and resources, leading to a feeling of powerlessness.

I have also felt alienated, because it is difficult to communicate this new perspective to medical colleagues. It is a challenge to describe my experience of seeing how, in my rheumatology patients, the mind and the body influence each other, without feeling unprofessional in some way. It remains difficult to prove, in biomedical terms, that I am having any benefit on disease. When the patient continues to worsen despite my best efforts and therapies, I have to confront the question of whether I am a failure as a MindBody clinician.

Helpful tools

I have found it pays to be able to slow down enough to recognize my thoughts, feelings and actions, if I want to make fundamental changes. This has been supported by adopting a reflective and embodied practice, such as mindfulness meditation (Grossman, Niemann, Schmidt, & Walach, 2004; Hofmann, Grossman, & Hinton, 2011). Writing a reflective diary and having regular supervision and personal psychotherapy sessions have all created space to allow for my personal growth. Being more self-aware, and consciously embodied, has helped recover and rehabilitate a part of myself that, quite frankly, was feeling stale and bored. Enjoyably, a curious depth to my thinking and understanding has developed, and now resides with me permanently. It has made me more open to the unknown and unexpected, and a tolerance of not knowing is growing.

The time and efficiency pressures in public teaching hospitals work against using the MindBody approach. I need to perform as well as I ever did, if not better, in diagnosing and treating illness from a biomedical perspective. The skill of combining the biomedical and the MindBody approaches develops over time, and the different emphases can be negotiated over several visits. Helpful and healing opportunities to discuss the meaning of disease will arise in the course of these sessions in a helpful way. I find educating patients about this is one of my tasks now. I have my own stories about how, when and why people have become ill, and recovered in response to a MindBody approach, and can use them as authentic examples. There are many patients where nothing has changed and the suffering is on-going.

My practice has changed to a more flexible interdisciplinary and pragmatic approach to patients and their illnesses, maintaining a quality of medical care, yet always remaining aware of what is happening beyond the medical version of events. Using the MindBody approach and being unskilled in psychotherapy has led me instead to collaborate with psychotherapists in the community. I share supervision sessions with them and we sometimes have shared patients.

It's a matter of judgment and skill to know when the MindBody approach will likely help, or when to use a purely biomedical approach mainly focused around medications. However, having a good relationship with the patient is paramount to both approaches, and so part of the skill is working hard not to alienate anyone. Thankfully, most patients welcome this approach. Because people are seen as individuals and not just as diagnoses, it is very rewarding relationally, and there is a dimension of fascination beyond that achieved with a purely diagnostic approach. One of the reasons people seek alternative or complementary medicine is their experience of the profound dualism in the biomedical system. The feedback from consumers has been mostly positive. I have presented my MindBody approach to rheumatology nurse specialists and arthritis patients with very positive responses, and, by request, to Arthritis New Zealand. Unfortunately, medical colleagues are often very sceptical, and I find this hard.

Aftershocks and re-building

The shifts keep happening. The transitions are on-going, and there has been an ever deepening transformation in my way of being and in my relationships with myself and my patients. It has not been merely the acquisition of a new clinical methodology. This earthquake has changed my personal and professional landscape.

At the end of the MindBody Course, at a time when I should have felt most pleased with myself, I wasn't. Instead I felt a great burden of having to integrate this new approach into rheumatology, and it simply wasn't happening. Interestingly, at this time, I developed an inflammatory arthritis myself. I had started to feel overwhelmed and unwell, and my hands became stuck. Ironically, I had to acquire my own rheumatologist who diagnosed rheumatoid arthritis. I have had to take my own medicine, literally speaking, and be patient with myself through this process of becoming a fully integrated MindBody practitioner, a process that requires me to be somewhat more compassionate towards myself. I had become overwhelmed by the burden of my patient's stories, unconscious and unprocessed, some of whom had potentially deadly diseases. Both I and my patients were stuck.

Incredibly, my body started to speak in a language that I had to listen to. This was another unexpected, disorientating and powerful aftershock, perhaps related to the new challenge of trying to be both a doctor and being put in the role of a person-centred psychotherapist. The end of the course was a signal for me that I was supposed to be accomplished and competent in this already, a very medical attitude. But the problem arose because whilst I had intellectually accepted this new paradigm, I had no training for the psychotherapy role, in fact I was out of touch emotionally. The emotional detachment required to be a doctor is definitely counter-productive to adopting a MindBody approach. I didn't want to stop being a rheumatologist and re-train as a psychotherapist, so the experience was exacting and difficult. It was quite a finale to the course, and perhaps a warning to other physicians planning on trying to change their paradigm. This may be a systemic barrier, arising from a healthcare system which has grown along the lines of dualism, to other physicians wanting to become integrated in their practice.

I feel very lucky to have another way of looking at what happened as a meaningful and potentially transformational experience. I feel fortunate to have avoided the disempowering experience of being diagnosed with a meaningless disease the way countless rheumatology patients have. More than that, I have discovered what I need in order to stay well, to be attentive to my own powerful emotions and not to be detached from them. In fact what is better than having a rheumatologist with personal experience of inflammatory arthritis and insight into how difficult it is to try and change their way of being.

Where to from here?

The aftershocks have subsided to some extent, and the re-building has started. I now acknowledge that the process of integrating the Mind-Body approach into my practice may take many years. It has required me to hold, in the same frame, the person's mind, body and spirit. I have an entirely new awareness of the relationship between the mind and the body in myself and in my patients. It has deconstructed my role as a doctor around diagnoses, targets and protocols, and reconstructed it with the person at the centre of care. I felt like I was sailing close to dangerous waters and no longer belonged in my medical community. By talking to my patients about their lives and what has affected them, my feeling for what is really going on, and what might be needed, has grown, and along with it my ability to bring healing. At the very least I can articulate this.

Developing my experience of the qualitative research methods needed to explore the phenomenon of the relations between life story and illness is one new direction for me. Phenomenological qualitative methods are ideally suited to researching the embodied life experience of individuals, and focussing on stress in autoimmune conditions with this methodology may be a way to bring the two worldviews together (Grbich, 1998; Husserl, 1967; Todres, 2007).

Being a member of the New Zealand MindBody Trust is another support structure and vehicle for progress. Building a community of like-minded individuals, fostering collegial relationships, consolidating my knowledge in my two new areas of ophthalmology and immunology, keeping engaged in supervision, perhaps developing my psychotherapy skills formally, and using mindfulness will all help. The soil is now more nutrient-rich and things are growing wildly. Finding a balance between all these new elements and potential directions, and staying healthy and present in the moment enough to enjoy my life, and being authentically myself, are now major priorities.

References

Brook, A. & Fenton, P. (1994). Psychological aspects of eye inflammation: a pilot research project. *The Psychiatrist, 18*: 135–137.

Broom, B. (2007). *Meaning-full disease. How personal experience and meanings cause and maintain physical illness.* London: Karnac.

Grbich, C. (1998). *Qualitative research in health: An introduction.* St Leonards, N. S. W: Allen & Unwin.

Griffith, J. L. & Elliot Griffith, M. (1994). *The body speaks: Therapeutic dialogues for mind-body problems.* New York: Basic Books.

Groddeck, G. (1932). Vision, the world of the eye and seeing without the eye. In: Groddeck, G. *The meaning of illness: selected psychoanalytic writings* (pp. 172–195). New York: International Universities Press, 1997.

Grossman, P., Niemann, L., Schmidt, S. & Walach, H. (2004). Mindfulness-based stress reduction and health benefits: A meta-analysis. *Journal of psychosomatic research, 57(1)*: 35–43.

Hofmann, S. G., Grossman, P., & Hinton, D. E. (2011). Loving-kindness and compassion meditation: Potential for psychological interventions. *Clinical psychology review, 31(7)*: 1126–1132.

Hoyt, T. S. M. (1957). *Psychosomatic ophthalmology.* Baltimore, MD: Williams and Wilkins.

Husserl, E. (Ed.). (1967). *Ideas: General introduction to phenomenology.* New York: Collier.

Jankovic, S., Raznatovic, M., Marinkovic, J., Maksimovic, N., Jankovic, J. & Djikanovic, B. (2009). Relevance of psychosomatic factors in psoriasis: a case-control study. *Acta Derm Venereol, 89(4)*: 364–368.

Stadter, M. (1996). *Object relations brief therapy: The therapeutic relationship in short-term work.* Northvale, NJ: Jason Aronson.

Thorne, D. M. B. (2007). *Person-centred counselling in action* (3rd ed.). London: Sage.

Todres, L. (2007). *Embodied enquiry.* Basingstoke, UK: Palgrave Macmillan.

Youngson, R. (2012). *Time to care.* Raglan: Rebelheart.

CHAPTER EIGHT

From fearing to caring: finding heart in nursing

Leeanne Ford

I have spent much of my career trying to find a way out of nursing, because my experience of it was mostly of fear and relentless doing. Moreover, I found it lonely, exhausting and very unsatisfying. I moved from workplace to workplace, in an attempt to find something different, not really sure what it was I was longing for, something deeply desired but unable to be articulated. Thus, here, I recount my journey towards integrating a MindBody and person-centred approach into nursing practice. I utilize very specific cases to illustrate this approach, and discuss how the process of embodying this is transforming my practice into a deeply fulfilling vocation that now holds value, meaning and purpose for me.

I was seventeen years old when I commenced my training. I met Mr. Sherman during my first summer break when I worked as an assistant nurse in a rest home. He was a big heavy man and a stroke had left him unable to speak, and one side of his body was paralyzed. Moving, showering, dressing, feeding, and cleaning him was hard work and physically tiring.

One day, while tidying the cupboard in his sparsely decorated room, I came across a photo of him taken when he was a young soldier, a handsome man wearing his uniform with both pride and humility in his face. Seeing the photograph jolted me, and I sank into a chair. Something opened for me, and for the grace of that opening I was present. All of a sudden, I was now able to see Mr. Sherman differently. I remember the frustration, sadness, fear and kindness in his deep dark eyes. I remember his big, soft, gentle hands. I felt a vulnerability that we both shared. I felt compassion.

My nursing training did not provide me with any understanding of what happened in that special moment, a moment which allowed a radically different perspective. It is through MindBody practices such as tai chi, mindfulness-based meditation, and study for a qualification in Mindbody Healthcare, that I now understand better what occurred in those moments with Mr. Sherman. I am able to attend to what is actually occurring, moment by moment, with patients.

I believe that on that day with Mr. Sherman I was able to be with the emotions in the room; his and mine. I was able to stay open to the "heart mind". Being with these emotions, just as they were, connected us.

In MindBody awareness even the space that we exist in becomes part of the experience of our interrelatedness. We become able to notice and empathize. In empathy, there is a deeper sensory responsiveness to the person, and, therefore, whilst I still had to feed, clean, shower and lift Mr. Sherman, the energy of these actions had a very different quality. This quality is, I believe, the heart of nursing.

My nursing training was grounded in a dualistic separation between mind, body and "heart"; in effect, the thinking mind became an entity capable of separateness from the heart. My training did not guide me on how to dwell in the "heart mind". In fact, I was mostly fearful when patients expressed deep emotion, and I certainly preferred to avoid them when they were doing so. I was not only fearful of my own capacity to handle emotions, but I also had a sense that there was little place in the healthcare system for the patients or myself to be human in the manner of deeply expressed and received emotions.

This dualistic approach has damaged nursing as a vocation, reducing it to regimens heavily governed by the importance of completing tasks and ticking boxes, and based fundamentally on a fear of getting things wrong. The nurse's fear of not adhering to the highly constrained and regulated aspects of any nursing regimen can tragically block a capacity for empathy. At the risk of sounding overly dramatic, this focus on adherence to nursing regimens in my training meant that I did not exist as a whole person in the nursing role, and I hardly had time for the patient to exist as a whole person. I believe that being trained in this way, as a young woman, failed me enormously.

I was burdened with the belief that a good nurse was one who completed tasks in a timely manner and without error. There was no guidance or encouragement to get to know my own inherent goodness and compassion. This same pattern was certainly reflected in the absence of any later professional development opportunities addressing these elements, and in my experience is typical of the entire nursing culture. I was left lonely, exhausted and defended.

Integrating a MindBody approach allows me to adhere to the practical tasks of any nursing regimen as part of the whole, but not as the whole. It has allowed me to place an appropriate emphasis on my own sense of personhood and that of others, including my patients and colleagues. Through MindBody philosophy, meditation, and mindfulness-based supervision I am becoming more open and increasingly aware of areas of my life contaminated by my nursing experience. I hope that now, rather than bowing to the fear of making a mistake (and the possible consequences of litigation and de-registration) and reacting by closing down to people, I would have the courage to accept my own humanness, and thus remain open, honest and available. The defensive position does not serve the patient or their family, nor does it serve me well.

This transformation has required me to be wholehearted. I have grappled with various philosophies, and I am learning to let go of deeply embedded views. I have stayed faithful to the process during times of utter confusion. I have been blessed with profound support from MindBody-based supervision, teachers and colleagues, which have been crucial in opening my mind to the reality of how things actually are; as they are. To be working this way changes nursing into a reciprocal, participatory, and meaningful craft.

My recent experience in the hospice environment has revealed that it is a person-centred approach that allows an awareness of the whole to emerge. It is from this work environment that I would like to share encounters that illuminate how a MindBody approach can be integrated into one's nursing practice. Indeed, more than that, they illuminate our everyday encounters with ourselves and others.

> The first encounter involved a patient who was admitted for control of her leg pain. In a duty handover I heard that Miss B had been

awake for the past three hours, and that the prescribed analgesia
had been administered, but with little effect. It had also been decided
that Miss B would be discharged the following day to her sister's
home in the South Island. I entered her room immediately after the
handover. Miss B explained that the pain in her leg had not eased
despite the medication she had received. I was immediately aware
of a warm and pulsating sensation in my hand, so I asked her if she
would like me to rub her leg. She agreed, and I stood massaging
her leg for about half an hour, during which time she said she was
comfortable. Apart from checking with her occasionally that the
hand pressure was good for her, few words were exchanged. I was
aware that Miss B's family were coming to take her home, and it
seemed this was very present with us as I massaged her. I simply
stated, "Your family is coming to take you home tomorrow." Her
eyes revealed her mixed feelings, and I felt these feelings with her.
We sat with them silently, until they seemed to dissipate naturally.
Her sister came to visit her, so we ended the massage with Miss B
declining the offer of more analgesic medications.

The dualistic perspective would assume that massaging this patient's
leg was simply just that; a nurse's hand massaging a patient's leg. From
a MindBody perspective however, it entailed a raft of micro-processes.
I was offering far more than just my hand. Miss B was offering far more
than just her leg. Our readiness to dwell in this place together allowed
an intimate union. Whilst we were two unique individuals, we were
also joined; in a way not separate. There seemed to be no helper and
no helped person, or a need for such categories. Rather, it seemed that,
in presence, our subtle relatedness joined us. We were open to connection, and willing to dwell in the space that we co-created. Halifax
(2009) asserts that this connection and openness are required to properly accompany a patient. Santorelli (2000) claims this union, in itself,
is healing.

The experience also served to decrease Miss B's pain levels. Dr. Cicely
Saunders (2006), founder of modern hospice care, conceptualized the
pain associated with the dying process as "total pain." She asserted
that total pain was tied to a sense of the person's story, and emphasized the importance of listening to the patient and of understanding
the experience of suffering in a multifaceted way. The act of stating that
Miss B would be leaving the hospice to go home served as a conduit

to summon the associated feelings inherent in her story. The act of us both allowing love, fear and death to reside in our space may have been instrumental in decreasing her pain level. Neuroscientist Rick Hanson (2009) says that the empathetic experience can be used to soothe, balance and even replace the negative story. He explains that the mind can hold the experience of the painful feelings along with the pleasant ones, such as the comfort of being understood and touched at the same time. Both experiences get infused, and in this case may have resulted in the decrease of pain experienced in her leg.

> I later returned to check on Miss B. As I was tidying up her room, I was looking for something else to serve as a connection for us. I noticed a prayer book on her table and said "you have a prayer book". I told her I loved to pray. She asked me if I believed in God. I answered with a certain conviction that I did, and added that I sometimes feel a sense of God. I noticed an expression of curiosity and a welcoming of further discussion. I sat down on the bed and asked her if she believed in God. She replied that she did but that she had never sensed God. She disclosed that she had experienced an encounter with an angel in her home one night. We chatted about this encounter and what it meant to her. She told me that people had doubted the validity of her experience and she was concerned what staff and relatives might think.

This encounter required mutual trust. I was prepared to disclose something of myself in order to connect with Miss B. Intuitively I used the prayer book as an invitation for connection. In the hospice, in particular, death is imminent. Miss B accepted the offer when she, in return, disclosed her experience and belief in angels. Disclosure requires trust and respect. Miss B and I both shared something from a tender place and we both met each other's experience with understanding and respect.

Within the hospice setting I see myself as a kind of midwife. The role of midwife involves the facilitation and accompaniment of the patient's transformation; in the hospice that transformation is death. In contrast with my experiences in other clinical settings, patients in the hospice seem to be more open to connection. This openness is both precursor and invitation to enter a precious, intimate space where the openness and connection continue. The nurse enables and holds this space where transformation is possible. Holding patients as they are, in those moments, gives them the space to transform if they need to. Thus we create safer openings, and possible passage, without forcing anything.

> One evening shift I was assigned to look after George, a sixty-three year old man. I had been told that his partner had decided that she could no longer care for him at home, and had found him a bed in a rest home. On entering his room I found him sitting on a chair, arms and legs crossed, his face red and tense. He was looking out the window. My immediate reaction was to try and soften his anger. I justified this by telling myself that anger does not benefit anyone, and that his life span was probably limited to a couple of weeks, and he might regret spending too much time angry at his spouse.

During supervision that week I reflected on this encounter. Eventually I realized I had recoiled from the anger, and shut down in fear. I had had no awareness of that fear and spent the rest of that shift with an agenda to get rid of his anger in an attempt to soothe my own discomfort. As a practitioner of mindfulness, I know that openness to whatever arises in the moment is what is required for healing. For whatever reason, I was unable to stay with what was present. My own fears around angry males had shut the door on connection with him. I could not open to what was presenting itself in this space. I had lost any capacity to hold the space for him.

Supervision and mindfulness practice have helped me to identify my own fear of anger. I have taken the opportunity to confront fear intimately. To be with it requires knowing it. Merleau-Ponty (1962) explains this as allowing the subjective experience to become objective. The objectification of the fear affords me the opportunity to create a space to observe the fear, and whatever arises in the space. This allows me to be open to whatever happens. In rejecting the anger, I was shutting down to what was present. In doing this I closed the door on authentic connection. Staying present with whatever arises is what is required.

In supervision I was also guided to shift the view I had on softening anger. I now see that my role is to soften to the anger. So whilst anger is present, my job is to remain soft and notice my tendency to tense in reaction to it. An intention to remain soft provides the platform to respond to what is required in the moment. I have taken the opportunity to consciously practice this with a lady who resides in a rest home that I also work in. She gets angry every morning when I give her tablets to her. I practice staying soft while she yells at me. Staying soft in this instance has a quality of firmness about it too. Whilst I soften to her anger, I remain firm in what I am there to do. This serves to hold the space rather than change it. Each time I have been able to do this, I get to witness a transformation.

> I met Bill, a forty-two year old Maori man two days before he died. I was assigned to care for him one evening shift. His level of consciousness was declining. He could no longer respond verbally and his eyes were now closed. I tended to Bill throughout the morning. After lunch some of his family members arrived. I entered the room to check on Bill and his family to see if anything was needed. I found Bill's wife, Rebecca, lugging her husband into a wheel chair. I was taken aback. Bill could not maintain a sitting position so I suggested a pillow to support him. I was privately hoping the pillow might also provide Bill with some comfort, as I was unsure how much pain he was experiencing. As Rebecca propelled the wheelchair forward she asked for directions to the north-facing veranda. I wondered if this request had something to do with Maori culture. Rebecca and her husband stayed outside for about one hour. When they were ready I assisted her to return him to bed. Rebecca and I washed her husband together. My approach with Bill was gentle. Rebecca's approach was brusque. As she was washing her husband, she was saying "it will be alright, hun", and "come on darl, lift up your arm, pull it through here." I continued with the gentle approach. Part way through sponging Bill, Rebecca began to soften. She said to me "Nursing must be so hard, I don't know how you all do it." I replied "Yes, it can be hard. It can also be really special."
>
> She sank down on to the bed and cried. She gently embraced her husband, stroking his face tenderly and telling him how much she loved him. Together, we finished washing Bill and did our best to make him comfortable in bed. Bill died two days later.

According to MindBody theory, presence is a powerful transformer. My presence in the encounter served as a model for Rebecca. Presence in a room has a contagious quality—despite this quality one has to recognize that people do not always have the capacity to encompass it. Empathy for this inability is what is required. Presence may have served as a mirror for care. In presence there is no judgment; this in itself can facilitate the transition.

Whilst New Zealand is very multicultural and it is necessary to acknowledge cultural differences, one does not want to be limited by culture. Approaching someone on the basis of their culture alone has the potential to discount the totality of personhood. Had I assumed that Rebecca's approach to her husband was culturally derived, the opportunity for me to model gentleness may not have occurred. A transformation from denial of Bill's condition and prognosis occurred in presence. The unique culture of the hospice environment places emphasis and focus on transition rather than cure. There is only limited technology available. When necessary, nurses remind patients and family that interventions are to relieve suffering, not to help someone get better. There are rules of safety in the health care system that cannot be disregarded. Whilst I may have assumed, from a safety perspective, that it was preferable for Bill to remain in his bed, it may not have been. It is probable that Rebecca would have had a better understanding of her husband's wishes. Because Bill was dressed and warm, and could not fall out of the wheelchair, he was safe. My own story of what constitutes a good death (in other words my agenda) could well have interfered with what turned out to be an important transition. My presence, in this situation, was to stay with my conflict around it and make sure he had a pillow. Preventing him from going to the garden would not have been a person-centred approach to safety. It would have been driven by my need to be technically correct from a procedural and safety perspective, but it would have been highly limited from a whole person perspective when, in the process of dying, an important goal is to let be and to let go (Dowling Singh, 1999).

Studying the MindBody approach and integrating this into practice requires much more than an engagement of one's intellect. It is essential that all of the faculties are engaged; mind, body, and spirit. In the hospice setting, MindBody interventions such as massage and an emphasis on connection are supported and encouraged. This focus on personhood requires openness to whatever is present. This approach of not knowing can, at times, be uncomfortable. However, my experience tells me it is very worthwhile. Through embracing a MindBody view, my perspective on illness, cure, and healing has changed. This change has afforded me a new and refreshing approach to nursing, which is rewarded with powerful experiences of myself and others as whole beings. They have served to bring meaning, value and purpose to my job as a nurse, and thus a return to nursing as a vocation.

Nursing training teaches us to do for, or to do to, a patient. A more integrated MindBody approach teaches us to be with a person. It redefines the relationship between the patient and nurse. This ability enables us to accompany the patient through whatever it is they are going through. This way of being with patients enriches the experience for the nurse and the patient and has positive health outcomes (Broom, 2011).

References

Broom, B. (2011). *Lecture notes.* AUT University MindBody Healthcare course.

Dowling Singh, K. (1999). *The grace in dying: how we are transformed spiritually as we die.* Dublin, Ireland: Newleaf.

Halifax, J. (2009). *Being with dying: cultivating compassion and fearlessness in the presence of death.* Boston, MA: Shambhala.

Hanson, R. (2009). *Buddhas's brain: the practical neuroscience of happiness, love and wisdom.* Oakland, CA: New Harbinger Publications, Inc.

Merleau-Ponty, M. (1962*). Phenomenology of perception.* New York: Routledge.

Santorelli, S. (2000). *Heal thy self.* New York: Random House.

Saunders, C. (2006). *Cicely Saunders: Selected writings 1958–2004.* New York: Oxford University Press.

CHAPTER NINE

Touching the hurt

Susan Lugton

M y special interest in touch and massage began when I was young. I remember experimenting with pressure and pain by pushing the sharp edge of a piece of Lego into the sole of my foot, and feeling the change from discomfort to a deeper pain. Then I would release the pressure and massage the hurt away. Sometimes in the evening, our family would form a "massage train" with Mother at the back massaging the shoulders of my sister or me, and Father, if he was lucky, sitting at the front, receiving a massage but not having to give one. My hands never tired of massaging, sessions often lasting through a one hour television programme.

These massage tendencies got me into trouble at a party when I was sixteen. Friends joked about the body language I was showing as I massaged quite naturally the shoulders of a boy in the group. I hastily dropped my hands; turning a deep shade of red (I do not remember liking the boy, but then again, perhaps my cheeks told another story). My close friends knew that I liked and was good at giving massages, and they would wriggle their shoulders in front of me, remarking their shoulders were sore. Touch seemed very natural to me. Instinctively, I knew it was both comforting and healing.

I was an enthusiastic, energetic and curious child, with a love of stories and their meanings. The Pollyanna books had a special place in my heart; that one could find a bright side in a difficult situation if dedicated to finding it. Her outlook influenced me throughout my childhood, as did the loving environment created by my parents. I loved listening to stories that my Mother or Aunt would tell at the beach when the weather was rainy and we were inside trying not to make too much noise. The other children would run off and play but I would prefer to sit and listen to the stories that emerged amidst laughter and cups of tea.

Furthermore, as a young child, I had a distinctive sense of posture and movement, knowing where my body was in space. From the age of six, I played the piano, sitting perfectly upright on the piano stool while I diligently practised. My regret during those years of piano playing was being too committed to the practice, rather than just playing for fun. I was to learn a very valuable lesson when sitting my grade eight Trinity piano examination at the age of sixteen. I made a decision to just play and not care how it went. I did not think I would pass, so I said to myself "what the heck!" I started playing with a passion that I had never felt before, my fingers running over the keyboard in a way that was deep with feeling and emotion. It felt great, feeling and hearing the music I was making. I had never played like this before. The moment I became aware of this I panicked and lost my place. When I finally began again, it was a far cry from the passionate playing I had surprised myself with moments earlier. Although I failed that exam by two marks, the comment from the examiner is one I will always remember; "I thought I was in for a musical treat and then you dried up on me completely." I did not care that I had failed, and in fact I was glad that I had. Most of my playing did not deserve the recognition of passing the grade eight Trinity Examination. Yet for those exquisite few moments, I played from the heart and the examiner noticed.

My mother was instrumental in pointing to physiotherapy as a fitting career for my personality and talents. There was an article written in the Waikato Times highlighting the role of physiotherapy in the rehabilitation of a young man who had been seriously mugged. The man described his eternal gratitude to the rehabilitation team for "getting him on his feet again" with particular reference to the young physiotherapist. She had worked skilfully and compassionately in helping him learn to walk again, and he expressed how significant she had been in his journey to becoming well. I distinctly remember being very moved by this story and decided there and then to be a physiotherapist. I was drawn to the relational component of his story, the patience and understanding needed to enable his rehabilitation journey.

I received a place in the 1989 physiotherapy student intake at Otago Polytechnic after re-telling this story to the intake interviewers, perhaps in itself revealing the power of stories to influence life's directions. I loved my three years of physiotherapy training. It was not so much the training as it was the personalities and enthusiasm of the bunch of students that learned with me. We oozed this love for life; active, dynamic, motivated and eager to learn. There are lots of training stories. I remember a particular anatomy lesson that involved marking the muscles of the shoulder on each other's skin. One of the men in the class was palpating my shoulder to mark the biceps tendon. A group of engineering students were walking past, only to stop short, press their noses to the window and mouth "What class are you in?" and "Can we join up?" After a very short time, bodies repeatedly marked, observed, assessed, analysed, and videoed, we became completely comfortable about exposing them to one another; although there was a mad rush to buy new underwear in those first few days.

Little did I know I was about to lose sight of stories and meanings in treating the person as I began this intensive three year training into the body as a predominantly biomedical, objective, and physical entity. The training was extensive. We learned anatomy, physiology, diagnosis, assessment tools, posture, palpation, movement patterns and function; but it was clinician-centred, led by objectivity and diagnosis with little value placed on subjectivity and the person. What little assessment of subjectivity there was, within this biomedical paradigm, left no room for feelings and personal story and was guided purely by the clinician. Over the years, as I attempted to learn more skills, clinical reasoning became the catch phrase. By the end of the history taking, it was deemed good clinical practice if you already had a clinical diagnosis that would then be merely confirmed or not by some form of objective assessment.

I became so focussed on getting the right diagnosis and fixing the problem I forgot to "touch the hurt." If the pain was in the buttock, pain sources could be lumber disc, somatic referral from higher lumbar joints, thoracic sympathetic referral, lumbar/hip instability, hip joint, or piriformis syndrome, to name a few. My mind was so full with all this biomedical information that I certainly didn't want a placebo effect disturbing my expert treatment.

As my skills at diagnosis became honed, my own feelings and understanding of myself and the other person became suppressed and ignored. I started to feel rather shackled as a physiotherapist, unable to bridge the divide between wishing to be properly relational with the person in front of me and hearing their story, whilst clinically diagnosing and treating her symptoms or disease condition. Much of this was unconscious, and I did not really understand what was going on. Feeling stressed and anxious, I could only put this down to not knowing enough, which drove me to further study. If I had understood that my anxiety and frustrations were highly meaningful and connected with my belief in the importance of treating the person, not just the condition or symptoms, my search for a whole person approach to healthcare might have begun earlier.

Early in my physiotherapy training, I spent two years in Vancouver, Canada, with a short stint in a neuro-rehabilitation hospital. Twice a week I would take the hydrotherapy classes for the stroke patients. One delightful gentleman would walk, with the help of his Zimmer frame, into the changing room sporting a bright green tee-shirt with the words "PARTY NAKED" splashed across his chest. It never ceased to get chuckles from the physiotherapy department. One day, as I was in the hydrotherapy pool with him, I stopped rehabilitating and started listening. He was telling me a story about his life as a fighter pilot in the First World War, meeting his wife-to-be on the ground after ejecting from his plane in a parachute. I remember thinking he sounded so young at heart. Just at that moment, he said, "You know, I don't feel ninety-one. I feel as if I could ask you out, and then I look down at my hands and realize I'm four generations too old." Upon reflection, that was the last time in that era that I recognized the importance of being relational with a patient.

Returning home to New Zealand, I felt this weight again on my shoulders to be the expert, trying to catch up to my peers who had completed the general hospital rotations as new graduates. I completely forgot to "relate and play" and enjoy my work. My intuitive skills for touch and massage were largely ignored and I was on the road to burn-out.

In 1997, I had a personal experience illustrating symbolically the MindBody connection. I was in my mid-twenties working in a busy London public hospital out-patients clinic. I had become completely entangled in a view of disease that focussed upon the body as physical, objective, and dysfunctional, expecting my knowledge of anatomy and joints to be able to fix the clinical presentations that walked through those doors, even if people had had symptoms for years. I internalized everything, nervous that I did not have the clinical skills to fix the patients, and I did not ask for help. My body started to vividly express my need for support. One day, after a particularly stressful day of treating patients with so many symptoms and issues, my right leg suddenly swelled up, like elephantiasis. After many biomedical investigations, I was diagnosed with benign lower leg lymphoedema, a condition affecting approximately ten per cent of young women. From an integrative perspective, I believe my lymphoedema was highly symbolic of my lived experiences and feelings around my work and expectations. Kovecses (2000) speaks of the shared metaphor across diverse cultures of "body as a container." This metaphor allows us to conceptualize intensity (filled with), control (contain) and loss of control (could not keep inside) (Kovecses, 2000). In my case, my body simply could not contain my internalized pressure and unconscious feelings of being unsupported any longer.

Returning to New Zealand, I followed a path of increasing my clinical reasoning knowledge, embarking on a postgraduate diploma in manipulative physiotherapy. On reflection, I was following in the footsteps of others who had completed this course; their reasoning and clinical understanding seemed far superior. Little did I know that I was searching for a true relationship with myself and the relational aspects of health-care. I was already operating out of a very cognitive headspace due to being anxious about getting "it" right, and the expert "fixing it", without recognizing that the patient needed some personal agency. The postgraduate course merely caused me to do more of the same. Following the course, I took on more responsibility for patients. Typically, I was treating patients every twenty minutes, with mounting stress levels, and I was so preoccupied with fixing the symptoms that I was, in effect, ignoring the person in front of me. I sensed other colleagues did not feel this anxiety, managing easily with these time frames, thus feeding my insecurities around my skill levels. After a patient made a complaint about becoming much worse after my treatment, I realized that I could not continue working in this sort of environment. In June 2000, with the advice of an older colleague, I decided to buy a practice that had a different approach. The colleague who established the practice recognized the importance of time, giving each patient at least forty-five minutes every session. Although I was nervous at going into private practice on my own, her philosophy made sense to me, and this allowed me some freedom to explore my own way.

In 2001, I had an encounter that was about to alter my life both personally and professionally. I had a delicious experience of learning how to breathe well with a physiotherapist, Tania Clifton-Smith, at Breathing Works, Auckland. I had organized the Breathing Works course for a number of physiotherapists as part of my role as the educational organizer for the Auckland Branch of the New Zealand Society of Physiotherapists. Tania had observed my breathing pattern over the day and suggested I would benefit seeing her individually. Tania embodied a sense of calm and grounded-ness within our session together that I had yearned for in my own career within physiotherapy. She was skilled, relational and inspiring, allowing me to rest in a peaceful place in my body and less in my head. I savoured every rise and fall of the diaphragm, enjoying every delicious moment of my body breathing for me. I remember thinking "this is gold." I felt grounded, calm and inspired that something so simple could have such a lasting and profound effect on me. It helped immensely in a personal way, settling my busy mind and providing a place of refuge when things seemed tricky or I felt anxious. I also found it extremely useful with the pain I experienced with endometriosis. When my monthly pain intensified I would lie down with a warm wheat bag on my belly and just breathe in and out mindfully, feeling my belly rise and fall gently. In minutes, my symptoms would melt away to a gentle ache giving me a real sense of the power of the breath. I learned to trust my breathing and the peacefulness and resilience it gave me if I tuned into it.

Learning to recognize breathing pattern disorders in my patients created a professional excitement that I had not previously found as a physiotherapist. Finally I had discovered a niche where I could slow down with my patients, creating an environment where they had permission to rest and be still with their body and symptoms. I grew to love teaching the breathing to patients because these sessions were the ones where they were the most delighted and grateful, frequently hopping off the bed and exclaiming they had never felt better or more relaxed. The breathing focus became invaluable to me as a practitioner, as my clinic began to draw more chronic pain patients with anxiety and often a complex array of other symptoms. I became more interested in the breath, reading books on mindfulness and breathing, and incorporating similar attitudes and techniques into my practice.

In 2007, I changed my business name to "Moving Well" wishing to illustrate the rich interplay I was observing between body, movement, breathing and mindfulness. My logo, although I did not quite realize it at the time, has become instrumental for my whole person approach. It is a circle of m's that become w's as you move around the circle; if you move, you are well and vice versa, conveying that our journeys are circular, forever evolving and dynamic. During my years as a physiotherapist I had observed a phenomenon that I fondly called "hurry sickness". People would arrive at my clinic in a fluster, presenting with pains and strains, frustrated at the untimely manner of their body becoming visible. Although the stories were always unique, there seemed to be themes of rushing, or "hurry sickness", around the time the symptoms appeared. I found this fascinating. People simply did not notice their bodies until they became painful and then when they did so their typical reactions were of anger, exasperation or frustration around the body playing up. I saw an opportunity to create an environment where people could come and experience their bodies in a different way.

Five years ago, I found myself in a personal situation that caused me to feel deeply anxious. I felt between "a rock and a hard place" and for the first time in my life, I could not be Pollyanna anymore. The levels of rawness and sadness emanating from that time have at times felt boundless, and at such times it has been difficult to see light at the end of the tunnel. The loss and grief were like a heavy cloak, configuring every thought, weighing down my heart. My breathing approach once again became my solace. It was reassuring, grounding, providing a break in my suffering as I drifted off to sleep. Journal writing became a morning ritual, softening my sadness as my deepest feelings formed into words. I stumbled on at work, struggling to be present with my patients' hurts when, as hard as I tried, I could not heal my own.

During this difficult time I had a chance encounter with an older family friend called Morrie, a lovely gentleman with a great sense of adventure and a youthful soul. Morrie gave me a wonderfully inspiring book called *Kitchen Table Wisdom*, by Rachel Naomi Remen (Remen, 1996), a physician specializing in psycho-oncology and a pioneer in training physicians in relationship-centred care. The stories she had collected over her life as a child, whilst training doctors, and from her patients, were deeply meaningful to me, re-igniting my excitement around the importance of being relational and compassionate with every patient encounter. I felt like I had come home. Finally, I was reading about the kind of healthcare that I wished to be involved in. These stories highlighted the importance of being present as an empathic witness, not afraid to show emotion, and able to accompany patients in their grief and sorrow, creating opportunities for healing. I also experienced a deeper sense of kindness and compassion towards myself when I was properly relational with my patients, although I did not quite understand the significance of this at the time. If I tried to remain business-like, and focus on diagnosis and treatment goals, I felt empty and exhausted. I struggled with the isolation of my own private practice, not recognizing that each and every patient who found their way to me was an opportunity for connection and relationship.

I took up a part-time position at the Hyperventilation Clinic at Auckland's Middlemore Hospital, to expand further into treating breathing disorders. The patients I saw at Middlemore came not only with a breathing disorder but also with deeply moving stories. I came to understand that telling me their stories, and having them listened to, changed their breathing more effectively than explaining the mechanics and physiology of diaphragmatic breathing. I was grateful no one questioned what went on in each hour because, for most of it, I would just listen. Intuitively, I felt their breathing disorders were symbolic of their suffering in some way and although I had the skills to alter their breathing pattern, it made sense to listen and try and understand why. I came to realize I was treating my patients in the same way Rachel Remen described, and it felt great.

A few months later, I attended an Accident Compensation Corporation physiotherapy meeting, and felt deeply disheartened that I was stuck in this world of physical outcome measures and functional goals with no space for relationship and connection. Overhearing my lament, a physiotherapy colleague, Lisa, previously unknown to me, turned and said, "You'd be interested in the MindBody papers at AUT University. It's all that you are talking about." I took the plunge, enrolled one week later and was to experience in that first weekend what I had been looking for all along. I was excited and enthusiastic about this learning. It seemed far less technical and mechanical than previous postgraduate papers, and opened up a world of philosophical ideas and questions about life and meaning. I was fascinated. I had always wondered whether I might leave physiotherapy and retrain as a psychologist, because I wished to be truly relational with patients rather than focusing on a painful body part. I knew psychology was not a good fit either, intuitively knowing that if someone was hurting, my natural instinct would be to reach out and touch; and I could not do that as a psychologist. Touch was one of my greatest assets. From a little girl, I had always understood the importance of it. I remember talking to Brian Broom before deciding to do the course. He said, "As a physiotherapist you are licensed to touch. That's an incredible privilege." I was not to know then, but embarking on the MindBody course would have a profound impact on my life. The greatest healing would not be with the patients I treated with this new philosophy, it would be within me.

During these two years, I came to recognize that peeling back the layers, although scary, created space for healing. A sort of renewal, like the feeling you get when you wake to a beautiful still morning, full with potential. Exploring my own sadness more deeply, I started to wonder about the meaning I had placed on my difficult personal experience, mentioned earlier. Sinking further into my feelings, a new understanding began to emerge. The greatest burden of all was beneath the grief and sadness. I had become so identified with my suffering that I could not let it go, as if it was now an essential and permanent part of me, and that letting it go would be tantamount to declaring that my experience was no longer meaningful or significant, when in truth it was sometimes as painful as it ever had been. But as I sat with this realisation, something started to evolve that had space and possibility. I recognized that in accepting my experience as part of me, it was also a gift, in that it created a deeper sense of understanding pain and suffering, and from this a wiser and more compassionate self emerged, with an ability to be imperfect and still whole.

I began to understand how it is to live with hurt and emotional pain, integrating this with optimism, hope, joy and excitement, and how real that is to those around you. My personal and professional life became blended into one. I was searching for the meaning in my experiences and although I had always put on a brave face during my clinical work, I gravitated towards letting my guard down and learning to feel what I was feeling, allowing my vulnerability to show. As difficult as that was, something incredible started to happen as I integrated my experiences and life story as a person. I began to experience a relationship with each of my patients, and for the first time in a long time, understood what had been missing in my earlier years as a physiotherapist, attempting to be the expert rather than drawing upon myself as a whole person, and connecting with another.

As I grew into my MindBody learning, I realized that searching for meaning, whether we are conscious of this or not, is why we are here. Each and every one of my patients who seeks treatment with me is a story, uniquely rich in experiences and deeper meanings. If we have not been heard, or feel misunderstood, often our emotional stories are expressed vividly in our body, for we are our body, and this may be the only way to truly represent what is going on for us (Chiozza, 1999; Merleau-Ponty, 1962). If we fail to understand this, and treat the aching body simply as a dysfunctional mechanical part, then we are saying that we need to be fixed, that we are broken, rather than appreciating that we are always whole, whether we are suffering or not. Merleau-Ponty, the French psychologist and philosopher, describes a "lived body" concept; that our body is our living interpreter of the world, and it is our body that perceives and overcomes the divide between the mental and the physical (Merleau-Ponty, 1962). This was a very different view of the body that I had learned about during physiotherapy training, and different to that of most of my patients. A former psychiatrist experiencing unrelenting buttock pain revealed her deep belief around the body as a vehicle: "It carries my mind around; that is all." Illustrating his mechanistic view of his body, another patient laments via a text message: "Su, I've broken down again. Can you fix me?"

Language and experience are heavily embedded in our bodies, providing a framework to understand how our personal stories can manifest as physical symptoms (Chiozza, 1999; Lakoff & Johnson, 1999). It is important to listen carefully to the specific language that patients' use, and to explore the often significant and revealing "off the cuff" comments. I now listen very intentionally to the words patients choose, because language is very often congruent with our life events, experience and reality in the world (Lakoff & Johnson, 1999).

> A patient suffering from acute bouts of vertigo and neck tightness described her desire to keep "on the right track" and on the "straight and narrow". I could not help but notice the interesting connections between this language of concreteness and rigidity that she used in describing her lived experiences both when growing up and

during medical training. Moreover, it was when she wavered from the right path that she experienced her vertigo. As we explored these ideas and feelings while I gently treated her neck, her vertigo symptoms abated.

Another example of embodiment appears with a patient presenting with an ankle sprain.

> One week prior to the ankle sprain, she described her ankle feeling "floppy, like a tooth about to come loose." I asked her what was going on around the time she experienced these sensations in her ankle. She replied she was "just holding things together", with four children home for the school holidays. I immediately noticed the symbolic link between the tenuous condition of her ankle and her tenuous coping as a mother. Listening to her language, I understood she needed support; both emotionally and physically. I provided the latter with ankle taping. Her symptoms settled during that session, which ended with her exclaiming that she felt herself again.

> A mother of three boisterous youngsters described her experience of three years of constant back and leg pain, which initially seemed to have no pattern. She said "I feel like I'm going around and around in circles." I noticed the exhaustion I felt listening to her story, and offered to her that we just stop going round in circles and see what happens to the symptoms. Tears welled up in her eyes, for my language was highly congruent with her experience of chasing her tail, running after her three boys with no chance of stopping. Her symptoms significantly improved after one session of teaching breathing techniques and slowing down, exploring the feelings around the constant juggling of motherhood.

Searching for meanings-related causes can shift symptoms and create healing.

> An illustrative example is Alice, an invalid beneficiary, who had experienced many hospital admissions for frightening "throat closing episodes." She required a CPAP machine to sleep at night and had a greatly diminished lifestyle to accommodate her shortage of breath. Medical professionals were perplexed by her presentation, exclaiming that her throat was "too small, too narrow,"

and consequently she felt ridiculed and invalidated. Listening to her language, I heard her words "I don't fit," primarily relating to being a buxom, flamboyant and creative woman in contrast to her other family members. This seemed to be echoed in some way when the medical professionals peered down her throat and described it as "too small, too narrow," perplexed as to how she could be like this. She spoke of not being able to voice her feelings during her relationships. No one had listened to her story. She carried around an adrenaline injection, despite medical opposition, and administered the adrenalin whenever she felt her throat closing over. I asked Alice if she was aware of any feelings or emotions at the time her throat began to close. She replied, "Oh no, it's totally a head response. I detach myself and simply watch from above." The significance of this sentence illustrates that Alice had become disconnected from her body, viewing it as an objective entity, and perpetuating the throat-closing symptoms when she did not feel heard. I made a conscious decision to listen to Alice's story. She elaborated with sketches of her lived experiences and after two sessions her sleep and chest pains had improved. To gently encourage connection between her mind and body, I took her through a mindfulness "body scan" on her third session to which she smiled, commenting, "I've never taken a trip down through my body before ... it is certainly playing up, isn't it?" Following these three sessions, and the experience of truly being heard, Alice went home the following day, opened her throat and sang like she had not done for years.

I was listening to the radio when the interviewer invited one of the oldest woman still working in the world, an Austrian psychotherapist, aged 102, to describe what she did. She replied, her voice full of patience, wrinkles and wisdom, "Oh, I just listen and try to understand the deeper layers beneath the story...." I pondered her simple words. It is about being relational and gentle, listening in a way that the person feels heard. That is how you touch their hurt. As Chiozza (1999) suggests, "merely fixing the symptoms does not heal the experience as the body finds another way to express unconscious story hiding in the body." Being heard is a powerful experience that needs to be understood as a fundamental human right and an integral part of every interaction between two people. Too often people are shut down, or their utterances glossed over as meaningless, even though the whole of the person is often represented in that very first encounter.

In conclusion, I bring myself as a person to my clinical encounters, meeting patients in a relational way, bringing a genuine interest towards their personhood and a healthy curiosity for what it is that brings them to me with their symptoms. As they begin telling their story, I attempt to listen intentionally to their words, their subjective experiences, observing their body and my own, noticing what emerges in the space that is playing out between us. I notice the feelings in the silences as much as the emotions that emerge with, and are implied by, the words; being an empathic witness to their stories. For so long I only focused on the physical, feeling the emotions hang in the room like a heavy curtain, unsure of how to acknowledge their presence or recognize their importance. Now I am comfortable with integrating language, emotions and experiences, exploring the potential connections between the body and mind. I have come full circle from that little girl experimenting with the Lego piece and placing my hands on others, to a physiotherapist who recognizes the deep need to be touched and heard. My days are filled with connection and authenticity. I realize that, as I have integrated the MindBody approach into my whole life, I do not feel alone anymore.

References

Chiozza, L. A. (1999). *Why do we fall ill?* Madison Connecticut: Psychosocial Press.

Kovecses, Z. (2000). *Metaphor and emotion.* Paris: Cambridge University Press.

Lakoff, G. & Johnson, M. (1999). *Philosophy in the flesh.* New York: Basic Books.

Merleau-Ponty, M. (1962). *Phenomenology of perception.* London: Routledge & Kegan Paul.

Remen, R. N. (1996). *Kitchen table wisdom.* Sydney: Pan Macmillan.

CHAPTER TEN

Issues in the tissues

Sharon Wood

Start on the hill
Glide all the way down, all the way to the end
Around the corner and back up the sheep's track
Send love through your hands and massage with your heart

—Penman 1995

This was my introduction to massage therapy eighteen years ago. In practice, it was a simple body map description of the relaxing stroke known as effleurage. Understanding its application would become easy, the hill was the iliac crest, all the way to the end was a full-handed connection with the erector spinae muscles, and back up the sheep's track meant contouring the sides of the body back to the waist. Send love through your hands and massage with your heart, seemingly simple words that would send me unknowingly on a journey of exploration, education, pain and healing to find my heart.

The search began with formal training in a diploma in therapeutic massage, followed by a diploma in clinical neuromuscular therapy and finally a bachelor's degree in health studies. Clinical work in multi-disciplinary settings followed, alongside opportunities in teaching, community promotion and presentations; even a television appearance. Personal healing occurred along the way, with attendance at a transformational healing course, use of body centred therapies, energy treatments and an exploration of my spirituality. Yet despite all of the above, the deep heart-centred connection I sought for my work and life remained distant. Three years ago, I felt disillusioned and despondent within both my practice and my teaching, and increasingly isolated within my profession. I was on the verge of leaving the industry when a colleague encouraged me to consider a course of study in MindBody Healthcare. This course ultimately transformed me and my practice through an understanding of what it means to be a unitary person.

The development of my practice towards a MindBody focus has at times been hugely challenging. I could understand the concepts intellectually, and I was very enthusiastic about the idea of expanding my clinical view to consider the multi-dimensional and multifactorial aspects of my clients. I began to see that somatic pain, movement difficulties and subjective story could all be operating in the same time and space; as expressions of the whole person. However, how does a massage therapist see, hear, sense and work with the bodily impressions of those stories?

The answers to those questions did not come easily and I grappled with many of the concepts for some time. Increasingly frustrated, I began to wonder if I needed to train in psychotherapy to be able to do this work. It had become apparent that not only did I have to assimilate, embody and incorporate new MindBody concepts into my practice but also, if I were to stay true to my hands-on profession and continue with touch as my core practice, I would have to re-evaluate the application and meanings of the many techniques that I had learnt. This required me to take some time out to reconsider my practice, and this could only happen by reflecting on my own story and my journey with massage to date.

Many times, I have been asked why I chose to be a massage therapist. The very simple answer is I never did. It just happened. It began with me experiencing massage in a beautiful way when my Plunket nurse (a New Zealand post-natal care service) taught me baby massage. Both my baby and I experienced a unified and loving communication. Keen to learn more, I attended a number of short courses that introduced me to the basics of Swedish massage. These weekend experiences unearthed a deep sense within me that massage was something very special.

I was invited to consider training for the Diploma in Therapeutic Massage but felt unsure about the study required. Anatomy, physiology and pathology seemed very daunting considering my unflattering science achievements at school. Yet, it was not the world of science that provided my first obstacle, but rather an invitation to reflect on my own personal healing philosophies. I was asked to consider the experiences and influences that had shaped me, and to notice how I had constructed belief systems around them, and how these might be influencing my decisions as a therapist.

My tutor modelled this request by telling us a story, a personal account of an early life experience that had influenced and shaped her future health beliefs and worldview. This was my first introduction to the concept that a person's subjective story could influence their health. I cannot remember all the details of the story, but I can remember how I felt hearing it. I admired the authenticity of the moment, it touched me; it took truth, courage and honesty, and I felt it very deeply. This was a transformational moment on two counts: first, I had just witnessed a true intimate healing moment and, second, I had just felt every word of that story in my own body and this frightened me.

Now it was my turn to try, and armed with my template I began to search for my own story. What would mine feel like, and could I be that authentic? I tried really hard, but I just could not connect with my past, my story, my heart. I couldn't feel anything and, especially, I could not feel my body. I was numb. This was deeply worrying and confusing. I could not then, or for the next fifteen years, find any words to describe this. The only way of coping I found was to try to push it away. I made a joke of it, supposing that even though I was only thirty years old this amnesia was definitely caused by menopause and it was just one of those things women go through.

Although I could not face my inner conflict at this time the exercise had made me realize that to be a good massage therapist (and I wanted to be one) I was going to need a lot more in my toolbox than just skilful rubbing. My challenge would be to blend the science and the heart-centred care and all that that embraced within my love for touch.

Working as a massage therapist in the early 1990s was certainly both interesting and challenging. Public interest in massage was growing and it was rapidly gaining popularity as a valid healthcare option. Massage is by no means a new therapy; in fact, it is recorded as being one of the oldest of the healing arts spanning across many cultures with references as far back as 500 BCE (Freeman, 2009).

In my early years of working, massage therapists in New Zealand had to contend with the stigma of the massage parlour industry. In fact, when I first qualified in order to work legally, I had to either declare myself under the Massage Parlours Act, or attach a rather long disclaimer to any advertising material stating that I was not practicing physiotherapy. Because of this, the formal training and education of massage therapists became essential and scientific principles available within the biomedical model provided a desirable professional framework.

Initially, being in the first wave of graduates who were biomedically trained was very exciting indeed. It seemed to generate goodwill and acceptance from other health professionals and opened up numerous employment opportunities especially within multidisciplinary healthcare clinics. My first opportunity came when I joined the team at my local osteopathic clinic.

Welcomed into the fold as the newly contracted relaxation massage therapist, I arrived armed with my sweet smelling oils and tranquil music. I could not wait to replicate what we had been practising in the classroom. In my training environment, our clients who were often referred to as "the body" would willingly quieten down, easily slip into a relaxed state and, quite often, the tranquil music was soon accompanied by deep vibrato snoring or even the dulcet tones of gentle purring. Unfortunately, my clinical experience did not reflect much of that. Mostly my clients found it extremely difficult to relax, were mostly restless, and seemed exceedingly talkative. Most disconcertingly, it felt like everyone I touched ended up in tears.

Amidst my efforts in trying to make sense of this phenomenon, I came to understand that the clients' talking, rather than being idle chit-chat, was mostly stories of their life experiences, and meaningful moments that had influenced and deeply affected their lives. Mostly the symptomatic physical presentations were back pain, headaches, or fatigue, but the subjective discussions were focussed on relationships, unresolved stresses, ill health, abuse, suicide and even death.

At that time, I understood the influence of caring massage, nurturing touch and therapist presence, and I knew I was creating a healing space for the subjective experiences to be shared, but I did not know how to hold this information together or navigate a healing path. I tried hard to find answers for them, but I had a dualistic understanding of a mind and a body, or, more specifically in my clinical situation, mental anguish and bodily pain. I reverted to my technical training, trying numerous bodywork techniques to fix my client's pain, but usually to no avail. Yet they kept returning week after week. I worried about their levels of distress.

I attempted to find answers but mentoring or supervisory support was difficult to find. There were only a few experienced massage therapists contactable, and, unfortunately, most of them were involved in a sports model of practice. In a clinical sense, I was on my own. Support from the Osteopathic team was limited. They too were not oriented to emotional material, and they strongly suggested to me that because I was purely a massage therapist emotional work was outside the scope of my practice. Massage training also supported this view. Greene and Goodrich-Dunn (2004) considered that the stimulation of the psychological aspect of the client was only a by-product of massage, not the central purpose. I was not intentionally making it a central purpose but it just kept happening. Without realizing it I was confronted by the Cartesian mind and body split (Leder, 1992) and its expression within Massage therapy.

This was an uncomfortable and confusing working space for me, but it did signal the beginning of my search for a therapeutic approach that recognized a unitary person. I began researching the influences of stress on people's health and looked for ways bodywork could help. Personally, I was getting very tired from the sessions. Unknowingly, I was empathically embodying people's experiences and this, combined with my unresolved body amnesia referred to above, led me to become unwell. I suspended working for a while and returned to further technique-based study. It seemed like a good time for a rest. I did not believe that there was anything wrong with me, probably just those broken ribs that I had when I was twelve, most likely exacerbated by my massage stance.

A difficult five years followed with a large list of personal health concerns that started to dominate my life, especially headaches and fatigue. I tried many practitioners for help, and was offered an array of diagnoses. Chronic tension headaches, trigger points, neuralgia, poor core strength, scoliosis imbalances, whiplash, a difficult birth process, food allergies, hormonal imbalances, thyroid deficiency, fibromyalgia and an autoimmune disease. Each consultation was essentially symptom-based and interventions were imposed on me that often made me feel guilty if they did not work. I began to wonder if any of this was real. It felt like nobody could see me, or hear what I was saying, even though I could describe my pain eloquently and vividly. I had a stabbing backache, and a relentless splitting headache. These were all words that fit well with some of my life experiences. Broom describes such language and meanings matching physical symptoms as somatic metaphors:

> (These are) apparent when a physical disease and/or its body location appears to be saying the same thing, expressing the same meaning as the patient's subjective "story," conveyed in verbal language or in the pattern of important and meaningful events in the life of the patient. (2002, p. 16)

This was a very lonely time for me. I had no certainty or even hope that I could get better. Eventually I surrendered to a pharmaceutical intervention, although I didn't want to do this. I felt less pleased when I was told that I could take these drugs indefinitely and that I would feel better. (Just pop back when I needed another prescription and good luck.) I left feeling so despondent. I felt like I had lost a battle, but who was it with?

Teaching a class one afternoon a colleague commented that I did not seem myself; "a bit dejected." She really listened as I relayed my story and finally I felt heard; she suggested that perhaps not all was lost and there were still some avenues I could explore. Rather than being relieved that finally I had been heard, I was furious. What other choices could I explore? Had I not been reaching out for answers for all these years? So I said to her: "If you tell me to go and find my heart, I am going to scream, because I don't have a clue what that means and nobody wants to tell me." I could see myself as the Tin Man, stiff, un-oiled and armoured, travelling along the yellow brick road trying to find my heart. The difference was that when the Tin Man searched for his heart he travelled with companions. I felt like I was travelling alone. Thankfully, this time I was not left alone and the support I received directed me onto a path of MindBody healing.

I was invited to attend an experiential day of Mindfulness, my first experience of healing presence. I started the day with no idea about what mindfulness was, and perhaps rather luckily I had no idea what the day's schedule was going to bring. This is how it went:

The facilitator gave us a raisin, with the simple instruction to "just be with the raisin."

My mind was racing. I had a headache and I remember thinking: "A raisin is going to stop my headache, you have got to be kidding, I'm out of here, this is nuts."

And then, looking around the room, I noticed that everyone was engrossed with their raisins, and I wanted to yell out: "Oh please, it's just a raisin. It's icky, look it's squishy and it smells."

Finally, there was another instruction, "put the raisin in your mouth, and just notice it."

Once again, I thought: "You must be joking! Thank goodness I didn't pay for this. Oh no, look at that lady over there, I think she is salivating."

But I did try, so I popped it in my mouth and said: "Ok, it's sweet, yep, makes your mouth salivary, there you go, swallowed it, all gone. Ok, all done, what's next?"

Unfortunately, for me the process went on and on and then finally some more instructions to "move it around in your mouth."

Now I was worried. "Oh no, I've swallowed it, what if they want it back, I've done it wrong, nobody else has swallowed theirs, oh well, what a stupid exercise anyway, how is this supposed to help my headache?"

This process dragged on for an extremely long twenty minutes. A group discussion and sharing about the experience followed, though I chose to alter and sanitize my story. Yet by listening and observing the other participants and quietly reflecting on what had really happened to me, I could see that each of us had just had a unique experience. Actually, it was enlightening to learn to just be with my headache without judging it. I began to understand that "healing requires receptivity and acceptance, a tuning to connectedness and wholeness" (Kabat-Zinn, 1996, p. 32). As the day ended, I had embraced the process and started to experience a deeper interior awareness, sensation and feeling. I was reconnecting with my body, myself and, yes, if you let it, healing can start by just noticing a raisin.

Participation in a number of healing and transformation courses followed, and I learned many MindBody techniques. My favourites involved imagery, colour and symbolism, and I found ways of expressing myself with pictures and images. Some of the early symbols remain powerful metaphors for me today. With a growing awareness of healing concepts and an ability to integrate some of these principles into my life, my body pain began to reduce and I started to work clinically again. I wanted to specialise in chronic pain conditions. It was only a matter of weeks before the earlier clinical experiences had repeated themselves again. The client's emotional upsets and stories resurfaced, and now I was convinced no amount of practical technique was ever going to be enough to meet these people's pain.

This was a conundrum for me because I had up-skilled and I was using and teaching advanced massage techniques. I had also tried to consider multi-factorial influences such as stress on bodily systems. Yet the recurring phenomena in my clinical work, and my own personal search for the felt sense of what it meant to "listen with your hands and massage with your heart" was enough for me to continue to seek answers, but this time within the framework of a MindBody approach.

I began my new study bemused by some of the words: unitary personhood, phenomenology, visible and invisible phenomena, embodied responses, and multiple realities. I learnt that the stories I had been hearing were expressions of my client's subjective experiences and clinically very important. The above terminologies revealed themselves as keys that could provide a healing framework that in turn could unearth the meanings. Blending and formulating these with bodywork proved difficult. With no pun intended, on the one hand I had philosophies that provided me with reason and verbal language skills, and on the other hand, I had touch. Singly they are both powerful healing agents, but I knew they could be more so if I could find a way to blend them together.

Studying the philosophical works of phenomenologists Husserl, Heidegger and Merleau-Ponty helped me to transform how I considered a body in practice. What was a body? I could draw on my biomedical experiences of componentry and working parts but the phenomenological concept suggested "the body as the primary context for experience and activity, thought and feeling" (Nathan, 1999, p. 198). This intrigued me. The term "lived body" was used to describe "where human thought, feeling, decision, experience, activity is lived out and such life is imprinted, sedimented, embodied, through each fibre of tissue" (Leder, 1992, p. 25). Nathan suggests that the tissues of the lived body are expressing their experience; "the patient's manner of living, therefore becomes also his manner of bodily being" (1999, p. 200). These powerful ideas were to unveil long sought-after answers to the felt sense, in myself and my clients, that our issues were in our tissues.

It was Leder's (1992) description of bodily experience as "intending entity" that helped to open my understanding of unitary connectedness. He used this term to describe the body's relationship with others, environments and the world. This suggested that "the lived body is not just one thing in the world, but a way in which the world comes to be" (p. 25). Slowly I began to understand and experience some of what it meant to be a living body myself, and work via the use of touch with another. I started to think about touch in different ways, how both my client and I would perceive touch and how collectively we would both give and receive. If I could adapt my clinical touch skills to work with a person in this way, a living and lived body, I knew I would start to feel and understand the meaning of "listening with your hands and massaging with your heart."

As alluded to earlier, massage is an ancient healing art. Tappan (1988) defines it as the "intentional and systematic manipulation of soft tissues of the body" (p. 3), suggesting it effects mechanical, physiological, reflexive and energetic changes. Influenced by the nineteenth century theories and applications of biomedicine and technology, new structural models of massage have emerged, my particular interests being Neuromuscular Therapy and Soft Tissue Therapy. Freeman says of these methods that they "seek to organize and integrate the body in relation to gravity, by manipulating the soft tissues or by correcting inappropriate patterns of movement" (2009, p. 365). In these instances, the use of touch is more of a manipulation-based intervention aligned closely with the Cartesian mechanical treatment focus. A lived body on the other hand would require a focus that utilized touch in a different way. Touch would become a form of communication providing listening and empathy and, in the safest sense of the word, intimacy. Ford (1999) discusses the communicative dimensions of touch and suggests that the qualities of touch can be more far-reaching than than just accessing pain or tension, capable of providing imagery and accessing feelings that relate to stored emotional experiences.

It is important to recognize the receptive qualities of the skin when discussing the qualities of touch. The skin is the oldest and the largest sensory system in the body, the most sensitive of our organs, our first medium of communication, and our most efficient protector (Montague, 1986). Our understanding of touch as a sensory input developing in the womb and continuing throughout our lives makes touch the first language of the body.

My first experiences of linking touch and MindBody happened unexpectedly. It was due to the acutely inflamed nature of a particular client's skin condition that I had to alter my repertoire of strokes and use of touch, and use touch to focus more on the receptivity of the skin. This enabled me to interpret the client's subjectivity in a different way, listen quietly, and use bodily sensations to help my client unfold and embody their own story. The difference in this approach was the allowing of time and space for the client's subjective story to emerge. It was as if we had started with a blank tablet, and because I did not, and in this case could not, impose any mechanical procedures on the presentation we just allowed the page to fill with the stories as they emerged. Then we could deepen into the felt experiences that were emerging and look for a connectedness that allowed a meaningful understanding to emerge for my client.

Working in this way continued to expand my ability to work with many clinical presentations. I have been working with people with depression, grief, skin conditions, irritable bowel disease, colitis, cancer, digestive complaints, and traumas. Many referrals happen by word of mouth and, at first, I found it a bit disconcerting that people were describing me as that healer who can remove emotions from the body, or, better still, "she does so much more than just massage." These are slightly scary words when you work in a field so commonly aligned to the sex industry. This highlighted for me the need to provide good educative processes for the clients and their communities; and the importance of on-going clinical discussions that keep reaffirming the collective and emergent processes of this work and especially acknowledging my role as a healing companion rather than a healer.

A clinical example involving a person dealing with the pain of a childhood trauma may help to show how touch and massage works within a MindBody framework, over a number of sessions. Traditionally, massage sessions begin with taking a health history and then a postural or movement analysis, and these remain essential to massage practice.

> In this particular client, the posture and movement patterns indicated muscular imbalances and tension patterns. While analysing the gravitational pulls I acknowledged the possible relations of this to physical, emotional, and storyfactors. I identified high muscle tonus and rigidity in the lumbar, thoracic and cervical regions where she seemed unable to feel or note any bodily sensations and

I had a "felt" sense she was not there, not in her body. Greene & Goodrich Dunn (2004) describes such bodily dissociation as a "form of disembodiment as a defence against feeling overwhelming pain or fear" (p. 129). By using a blend of verbal dialogue and non-verbal touch, her story began to unfold. She identified two powerful wishes, first, to "just feel happy again" and second, a heartfelt request to please "help me get 'it' out of my body." In all senses of the word it was a touching case.

In an attempt to work with the dissociation, or ungrounded aspect, I tried numerous touch techniques such as relaxation massage, energetic holds on and off the body, soft tissue and neuromuscular therapies, but mostly they remained ineffective. Whilst doing this, we talked about the story aspects of her life. This would be initiated by the client and would always begin in response to a feeling or sensation that she was noticing in the session. At times, it would seem like a game of back and forth waiting for an opening to appear. This was difficult for me. My training had taught me to seek only one truth, test it and then use a soft tissue intervention to fix it. Now I was asking myself to extend what Husserl refers to as my "natural attitude" (Sokolowski, 1999) to question what I see, what I allow myself to see, and to what extent am I willing to look at wider and multiple realities.

This required me to be open to whatever phenomena that might present, and trust in the process and myself. I needed to work very hard to quieten my own fearful thoughts, and to extend my own presence, changing from an empathetic to an intimate stance, an intimacy that could provide a safe holding space and would allow her an opportunity to release or reveal deep subjectivity.

We did get to such a moment. I used the non-verbal qualities of touch to communicate and provide safety throughout the process. One hand listened intuitively for feedback on her comfort and tolerance levels, whilst sensing the unfolding story. I remained attuned to her feelings, especially her fear, anger and sadness. At times, I had glimpses of important life events. The other hand offered support with safe contact by using a variety of pressures and placements to provide comfort and presence. As the process deepened, her breathing would intensify and she would begin to shake, releasing silent tears. Sometimes her body would convulse. These processes typically continued in waves for approximately half an hour before a settling period and then calm, and after some silence, she commented, "You are the first person that I know who really understands how I feel" and then "I didn't want to be in my body, it was such a scary place to be." In this very connected moment we were able to bring together a number of experiences that were pivotal to the understanding and meaning that my client had been seeking within her healing process.

The approach used with this client was both personal and individually tailored to suit her. This is the aspect I enjoy most about the MindBody philosophy. Each person is unique. I found that working with physical and subjective experiences did not mean that I had to forgo my previous skill set but rather adapt and broaden my view of massage and touch. This in itself was a gift. I am in awe of the healing power of touch within a MindBody healing framework.

My professional and personal search for meaning has spanned nearly twenty years and many of the jigsaw pieces are now in view and interlocking. I can see now that the concept of story has been an integral part of this journey. Dealing with my clients' micro stories has revealed aspects of my own truth. Early on there was difficulty listening for and hearing the client stories. I was challenged into a deep personal development as a clinician, arising from the frightening reality that I could not connect with my own story. Mostly stories are revealed in words, but I could not find the words, any words. Then I learned that the words themselves were not that important, it was how I felt, and how I experienced, and how I embodied my own story that was important; this enabled me to then be with my clients in both a new and unitary way. I am grateful for the learning I gained from the MindBody framework; that, when combined with the very caring holding of some supervisors and healing companions along the way, it enabled me to open up to a world of rich multi-dimensional realities. It has been a lengthy learning process but a deeply felt one and now I can honestly say that I understand, embrace, and embody what it means to "send love through your hands and massage with your heart."

References

Broom, B. (2002). Somatic metaphor: A clinical phenomenon pointing to a new model of disease, personhood, and physical reality. *Advances in Mind/Body Medicine, 18*: 16–29.

Greene, E. & Goodrich-Dunn, B. (2004). *The Psychology of the body*. Baltimore, MD: Lippincott Williams & Wilkins.

Ford, C. (1999). *Compassionate touch: the body's role in emotional healing and recovery*. Berkeley, CA: North Atlantic.

Freeman, L. (2009). *Mosby's complementary & alternative medicine. A research based approach* (3rd ed.). St Louis, MO: Elsevier.

Kabat-Zinn, J. (1996). *Full catastrophe living: how to cope with stress, pain and illness using mindfulness meditation* (15th anniversary ed.). New York: Bantam.

Leder, D. (1992). A Tale of two bodies: the cartesian corpse and the lived body. In: D. Leder (Ed.), *The body in medical thought and practice* (pp. 17–35). London: Kluwer Academic.

Montague, A. (1986). *Touching: the human significance of the skin* (3rd ed.). New York: Harper & Row.

Nathan, B. (1999). *Touch and emotion in manual therapy*. London: Harcourt Brace.

Penman, S. (1995). Personal communication.

Sokolowski, R. (1999). Husserl, Edmund. In: R. Audi (Ed.), *The Cambridge dictionary of philosophy* (2nd ed.) (p. 406). Cambridge, UK: Cambridge University Press.

Tappan, F. (1988). *Healing massage techniques*. Connecticut: Appleton & Lange.

CHAPTER ELEVEN

There is always "something else": phenomenological physiotherapy

Julian Cloete

"I've lost my power"

Lois presented with a tennis elbow. Elbow problems are often symbolic of overcompensation for some dysfunction in another part of the body, perhaps the hand or even the shoulder. In Lois's case there were a few issues with her shoulder, but treatment and exercise over a couple of weeks did not have the desired effect. She noted that her elbow was worse at work, especially if she was under a lot of stress. We chatted about the time when the injury started, and she mentioned that preceding the injury she had experienced a loss of power in her tennis serve and forearm shots. "Hmm," I thought, "a loss of power is a meaning that fits this physical problem." Interestingly, in her work, her employees were letting her down, and she was struggling to control the direction of her business. When talking about these issues she seemed to lose her usual confidence and energy; lacking "oomph," as she called it. When I worked on her shoulder and arm, I became aware of my own embodied sense of resignation and loss of power.

I often let things stew inside me for a few minutes to develop a better sense of what I am seeing. As Lois talked, I felt a sense of resignation, and when I became more secure in this feeling I asked if she felt a general loss of control, to which she responded, "Yes I have lost my power." It all fell into place for her how her injuries and work issues were related. Through hard work, dedication and energy she had built up her business, but some employees were just tagging along and not investing themselves, and she felt powerless. She knew she had to make some big decisions but had been delaying these. She developed a sense of how this was affecting her as a whole, and began to imagine finding a way to get her power back.

Lois's elbow pain has improved significantly and she continues to make decisions about the future of her business. She is regaining her power, and who knows what the next tennis season may bring.

Reasons, meanings, touch, talk and boundary-riding

Over the last couple of years I have become convinced that everything happens for a reason. I often ask my patients, "If, for some strange reason, everything happens for a reason, I wonder what reasons could be behind what is happening to you?" This is done with a neutral but genuine curiosity, giving the patient time to respond, even if at first they say they do not know. In my experience, the actual answers given are not as surprising as the matter-of-fact way in which the answers are often conveyed; as if the reason is strikingly evident.

I have always enjoyed being a hands-on physiotherapist and find it very satisfying to help a person feel better, both physically and mentally. To me, the physical, mental, and emotional dimensions of well-being are inseparable. Pain and physical problems bring about challenges that often require change in both body and mind so that healing can take place. The more I am open to this the more it confirms itself. Finding the reasons and meanings behind injury and pain, with and for my patients, is a way of enjoying the rich flavours of life as they emerge in my daily clinical work.

The dualistic construction of medicine steers us to either "talk therapies" or "touch therapies," and professional boundaries are constructed to confine us accordingly. In this chapter, I will explore the touch/talk boundary, seeing it not as a well-defined line, but rather as a vast no-man's land, where psychotherapy knowledge and experience and touch therapy merge.

Something else is going on!

In my early years as a physiotherapist working with chronic pain patients, I was frequently aware that something else was going on. I could see that some patients' problems (and pain) lay outside the physical dimension of health, even though the symptoms were overtly physical in nature. I instinctively knew there was something else, but it was elusive, and it started me on my journey of looking beyond the body and physical medicine.

I was often frustrated by patients presenting with pain where psychosocial factors were clearly contributing, and I would suggest that they needed to see someone (perhaps a psychologist) to discuss those issues. Patients would often react by saying: "Can't you help me?" or "can't I talk to you?" They felt this way not only because we had built up rapport and trust, but also because I had acknowledged them as whole persons, and their problem as part of a whole picture. I had usually established a trustworthy intimate connection, at least partly helped by treatments involving touch. I would remind them that I was not qualified or trained. I felt limited both by my perceived lack of professional skills, and by professional boundaries. I have subsequently learned this was wrong in a number of important ways.

Who am I in the therapeutic space?

Fundamentally, as a person, I am already positioned and potentially able to meet my patients on a personal level and engage in a therapeutic relationship. I have learned to let go of the confines of the biomedical model and the restrained, distant stance of the all-knowing professional who does not get personally involved. When I am in a session with a patient, we are two people, and we are two specialists. I am the specialist with my toolbox of physiotherapy skills and the patient is the specialist of him or herself. At that moment, no one knows patients better than themselves, and they direct me to which tool I should use to help them. I have the experience on how to use the tool needed, and through using that tool, I become personally involved with my patient. As a professional, this personal involvement is short-lived; when patients leave, not only do I have to let them go physically, but I also need to let go of my experience with them and not carry their burdens. I will discuss this later from the perspective of reflection and supervision.

I am not saying that I am a physiotherapist who can engage in psychotherapy with a patient. I still refer people with overt and complex psychological problems to appropriate professionals. My talk therapy with a patient is perhaps analogous to a psychotherapist massaging an anxious patient's tight shoulders. The psychotherapist might provide some relief, but would not be able to treat the patient's rotator cuff impingement. Not that many psychotherapists would offer such massage, because the issue of touch in psychotherapy is very contentious. As a manual therapist, professionally entitled to both touch and talk, I have a huge opportunity to help my patients. I will explore this later under embodied counter-transference.

Trapped in my paradigm

As a physiotherapist straight out of university, my paradigm or worldview, that systematic structuring of what I knew to be true and possible, was limited. I tended to reject things, often subconsciously, that did not fit into my paradigm. I could not, for instance, accommodate the view that emotions and thoughts can elicit a physical response such as inflammation in the body, a stance typical of the reductionist attitudes underpinning most of modern medicine. Although quantitative scientific investigation has led us to some amazing advances in medicine, I have realized that expanding my view beyond the entrenched mono-realities of reductionism is the way forward (Nicholls & Gibson, 2010). I now adopt the multiple-reality view of postmodernism (Grant & Giddings, 2002). Opening up my world view has allowed me to do the things I do better. I have not learned any new treatment techniques or methods, just a better way of using them, because I interpret situations differently.

The marriage of the reductionist attitude with evidence-based medicine has led to a "just one way" ethos. When one proves that a type of treatment works well, buttressed with good evidence, reductionist minds tend to conclude that no other type of treatment could be as effective. I agree with the aim of evidence-based medicine to show what works, but I try to be aware of other possibilities too.

There is growing understanding in physiotherapy that the biomechanical approach is inadequate (Overmeer, Boersma, Main & Linton, 2009), that physiotherapists need to treat their patients as unique individuals (Edwards & Richardson, 2008), and that the data of evidence-based medicine, based on the treatment of groups, does not take into account the unique individual. Our education system needs to embrace and reinforce that there are usually many ways to treat problems. If students are not taught to keep their options open, they fall into a routine of doing what is thought to work best most of the time, a safe route for the clinician perhaps but one that tends to minimize presence and personality. It is not geared to treating patients as individuals. I have made this mistake.

More than just a "physio"

My first experiences of holistic treatment were distinctly biomechanical. I discovered, under the guidance of my first employer, that physical problems in a part of the body (for example, the knee) could be caused by dysfunction of another part (for example, the hip and pelvis). Simply put, a movement problem in a patient's hips could cause knee pain through overcompensation. I became concerned for looking at the bigger picture. What I did not realize at that time was how big the picture is.

I also became very aware of the body's innate ability to heal. The important point was that the knee problem was due to something else (the hip in this instance). This naturally led me to the idea that when an injury was not healing as we would expect it to, there must be another element, that elusive something else, causing conflict in the body. This was really the start of my quest to find the stuck bit, and address that, so that the body could then continue to heal.

I also noticed that a particular hip and pelvis problem may cause left knee pain in one patient and right foot pain in the next patient. So everyone is different, and I learned not to presume things or generalize so much. Exploring the unique individuality of each patient gave me tremendous job satisfaction, because two injuries were never the same. This had a very helpful indirect effect, because my patients often felt I was particularly interested in them, which made it easy to build rapport.

I still maintain a strong interest in biomechanics and the way we move. Sports people talk about the effortlessness they experience when they are in the zone. This, to me, is the epitome of smart work by the body. However, our thoughts, emotions and states of mind also affect our movement and biomechanics. Sometimes we can feel right on top of things physically, then everything suddenly falls apart emotionally, and the body sags commensurately. Aha, the picture just gets a whole lot bigger.

Hold on—things are getting out of control

I was not skilled enough to manage the bigger picture. At one stage I felt I should study psychology. At other times, I felt let down that there had been no practical psychology in my undergraduate education, nor any whole person-oriented supervision in my physiotherapy training. For most physiotherapists, a supervisor is a colleague who has more knowledge, experience and skills than you and will be a type of teacher or leader; basically, a better physiotherapist. Sometimes supervision happens informally, perhaps the commonest example being the tea room rhetoric about a difficult patient, which I have often witnessed in physiotherapy clinics. However, in psychotherapy, supervision is where the clinician can discuss and debrief their own issues, experiences and feelings regarding their work. It is about your process, and working through that. A supervisor is frequently someone more experienced, but all supervisors bring another set of eyes and ears and a degree of accountability to one's practice. I have found this type of process supervision invaluable in my growth as a holistic physiotherapist.

There is a fair amount of literature calling for more supervision and reflexivity in physiotherapy training (Edwards & Richardson, 2008; Gibson, Nixon & Nicholls, 2010; Nicholls & Gibson, 2010). Reflexivity is the practice of self-reflection about our experiences in clinical practice. This has a more subjective focus than the "did I do the correct treatment?" question, which the "just one way" approach fosters. I do not find reflexivity to be an easy process, as it tends to expose my faults and weaknesses and sometimes leaves me feeling vulnerable. However, the personal growth and self-confidence I have gained are very rewarding. There is something enlightening and empowering about conquering my own fears and inadequacies.

Phenomenological clinical reasoning

As a physiotherapist, I do indeed work outside the square, but I also have high regard for being a proficient physiotherapist in orthodox terms. I strive to do the basics right, and good clinical reasoning is an important part of this. Clinical reasoning is derived from a hypothetic-deductive process in which I use the patient's symptoms and signs to develop a diagnosis, and indicate applicable treatment (Edwards & Richardson, 2008). This reasoning demonstrates that I understand the injury in detail, according to orthodox patterns of understanding, which then empowers me to do specific and effective treatment. Clinical reasoning also requires me to be able to differentiate between different injuries with similar symptoms. As normally practised, clinical reasoning is often highly reductive, but it has value, is easily taught, and, as it happens, can be enhanced to accommodate a whole person approach. The physical body, with its relative measurability and predictability, does still fit well with a reductionist paradigm. We all have two arms, internal organs, and similar physiologies. However, as soon as we consider the person as a whole, a more post-modern view is necessary. Two bodies are very similar, two people are not.

The method behind clinical reasoning is to interview a patient about their symptoms and history, probing for objective clues while filtering out the noise of subjectivity. The trap is that, if I follow this reasoning process, I only understand the patient according to the reductionist paradigm of physical injury; for example, that the patient's back pain is from a strained muscle, but not necessarily all the reasons why the muscle has given in under the strain. Frequently, symptoms do not fit a pattern or make sense for a specific injury, and, furthermore, patients' responses to apparently similar injuries differ greatly.

The concept of phenomenology, the unique lived experience of a person, and how that experience will differ from one person to the next, has enabled exploration and illumination of these issues and clinical situations (Sokolowski, 2000). A person who hurts their back and cannot go to work for a few days will have a different experience from another person with a similar sore back who cannot play with their children. I have learned to nurture a phenomenological attitude, which involves bracketing or suspending my preconceptions (Wertz, 2005). This means that, momentarily and relatively-speaking, I put aside my experience and worldview and see a patient's problems through their eyes or experience. This gives me a better understanding of the patient's lived experience. The phenomenological attitude has profoundly affected my clinical reasoning skills but it has taken time and effort to develop. Bion and Freud (cited in Feldman, 2007) remind me that I need to be careful of prejudging my patients' experiences, and finding what I already know. This means being present and open to the patients' experiences as they unfold during therapy. In other words, I need to really listen to what my patients tell me, and how they do so.

A patient will make sense of the meaning that an injury or a pain holds for them through language, posture and even body gestures (Finlay, 2006). So when a patient says "my back pain is really awful; it feels like my back is going to give way", I ask them to elaborate on the feeling of giving way and try to understand what that means to them, or why it feels so awful. The exact words a patient uses hold clues to their experience. It can be that simple, yet truly deep and meaningful.

I confess to relishing clinical reasoning because it allows me to play detective with respect to diagnosis. Now there is something else. When I also deploy the phenomenological attitude, I gain insight into my patients' experiences and even their expectations. So, I start with a post-modern attitude of anything is possible, of openness to multiple levels, and then let the patient tell their story. When I interview a patient, I think of starting with a blank sheet or a net. As the patient tells their story, my conscious net catches the important things. Yes, I am still listening for physical symptoms to generate a physical diagnosis, to do the basics right. Yet I am also picking up other nuggets of information. I am trying to capture the patient's lived experience. This in turn helps the patient feel heard and therefore more open to the process. The beauty of this method is that when the symptoms do not make sense in a reductionist way, I will already have gathered other information about their experience; meaning dimensions emerge, and I will be a step closer in helping that patient find meaning in their problems. A good example of this is fibromyalgia where the patient's experience of physical pain is very real, yet there is often a lack of physical explanation or observable pathological process. With such a patient, I have found their story is often very meaningful. From a post-modern perspective, all symptoms make sense to me on some level. The manner in which I try and understand the patient's symptoms and story concurrently is what I call phenomenological clinical reasoning. It can be phenomenal.

Putting the "therapy" back into "physio"

I feel the physical closeness engendered by touch creates a context allowing benefits for my patient beyond just physical help. Touching and talking allow a rich therapeutic space, which includes all aspects of interaction between my patient and me. In the intersubjective relationship of therapy, both of us are present as people. We each bring our histories and our entire embodied selves. According to Soth, (cited in Totton, 2005) as we start to interact our inner worlds become interwoven and enmeshed. This means I cannot separate myself from a therapeutic relationship and just be the professional. I have to engage with my patients on a personal level. I have found that an understanding of a patient's transference to me, and my counter-transference in response, is something else to consider and utilize in the cause of good treatment.

A patient's internal world, especially repressions and conflicts, manifested in their transference, are projected towards me as the clinician "other" in the relationship (Feldman, 2007). Samuel, (cited in Stone, 2006) explains counter-transference as the reactions in the therapist's inner world in response to the transference projections of the patient's inner world. Put simply, counter-transference comprises the specific emotional responses aroused in the therapist by specific qualities of his or her patient (Ross, 2000).

I treated two very different patients in whom understanding transference and counter-transference proved very useful. With both of them, I felt frustrated and unsure of what I was doing wrong, because both patients' injuries were taking longer than expected to heal. I knew my treatment should be effective and I could not think of anything I should be doing differently. It was then that I considered I might be picking up on my patients' frustrations. Each patient was feeling frustrated by more than just their injury; and that was their transference. My counter-transference was the frustration that I was feeling as a consequence. I raised this issue of frustration with both patients, initially only about their injuries, but it did not take much invitation for them to spill over and vent their current frustrations in life. The process of acknowledging their frustrations was enough to help them move forward. Working through the frustrations seemed to clear the air for my patients and their injuries then healed as expected. Transference and counter-transference is happening all the time, and being aware of it helps me understand not only my patients' lived experiences, but also their needs. It also helps me, as a physiotherapist, with my own reflection and growth. This in turn creates a better therapeutic space where my patients can more comfortably express themselves, giving me more to work with.

I also notice in myself the tension between being a "good physio" doing the "right things" and being a "holistic therapist" who is prepared to look for the "something else." It is almost as if I have to embrace the dualistic split of doing the "correct treatment biomechanically" and being a caring individual with a holistic approach.

Embodied countertransference

The meaning of "embodiment"

Merleau-Ponty (cited in Finlay, 2006, p. 19) said: "The body is the vehicle of being in the world" and "I am my body." Our bodies connect us to the world, and allow us to understand ourselves and others. Finlay (2006) offers a poignant personal example. She worked with a patient who had decreased sensation in her hand. Medically, it meant her function was impaired by the diminished ability to feel the difference between objects or textures. This medical description is sterile compared to the patient's subjective experience of not being able to feel the softness of her baby's skin and, in this way, diminishing her connection as a mother. That sinking feeling in my (and your) heart right now is as embodied as is possible.

Being aware of my embodiment, both physically and emotionally, helps me to connect to my patients and treat their problems in the best way I can. It gives me clues to the unseen signs and symptoms, and to the richness and depth of my patients' experiences of their problems. Phenomenologically, their experiences and actual pain are entangled and inseparable anyway. It is useful and meaningful for me to see and feel the whole picture when working with a patient.

Mirrored in science

Modern neuroscience and functional MRIs have provided some insight into intersubjectivity and human interaction. The science behind transference and counter-transference is described by Gallese (2009) as embodied simulation through mirror neurons that have been discovered in the brain. Our interactions with other people are both mirrored and embodied, whether we are aware of it or not. My aim is to learn to be receptive to embodied counter-transference and to use it as a tool to help my patients. Gallese cites a large number of studies showing that mirror neurons are linked in sharing of emotions, touch sensations and pain perceptions. Eureka! It seems there is scientific evidence of my experience; that we can truly share an embodied simulation of another person's real experience.

Now back to touch, gently:

> In order to use your hands and begin to develop them as reliable instruments for diagnosis and treatment, you must learn to trust them and the information they can give you. Learning to trust your hands is not an easy task. You must learn to shut off your conscious, critical mind while you palpate for subtle changes in the body you are examining. You must adopt the empirical attitude so that you may temporarily accept *without question* those perceptions which come into your brain from your hands. Although this attitude is unpalatable to most scientists, it is recommended that you give it a short trial. (Upledger, 1983, p. 26)

In my journey exploring the body and mind I have tried many different approaches. The work of John Upledger (Craniosacral therapy) and Jean Pierre Barral (Visceral Manipulation) have been most influential with respect to the touch side of my therapies. Both use very gentle physical touch to help bring about change in a patient's body and to promote healing. I subscribe very strongly to helping the body heal itself. Upledger's words (vide supra) will likely bring a smile to the face of many phenomenologists. Phenomenology reminds me to suspend my judgment in order to understand my patient's experience (Sokolowski, 2000). By working in this touching, gentle and receptive way, I can allow the body to express its problems (Barral, 1996). It then comes down to what I do with what I feel.

Reflections on my work experience

In pursuing the "something else", a number of surprising, yet in the end not so surprising, dimensions and concepts have guided my growth as a MindBody physiotherapist. The picture is now much bigger. When I am working with patients, the first step is to trust myself and be open to a wider and deeper process of understanding my patients' experiences. It might take time and I need to stay open and curious, but not judgmental. I am receptive to what I feel in their bodies, hear in their words

and see in their movements or postures. I find both regular meditation and physical exercise very helpful for this. I am conscious that the
feelings I embody often mean something different to my patients than
they do to me. I try to recognize what "my stuff" is, which minimizes
the possibility of me projecting this onto my patients. I say minimize
because once I enter the intersubjective relationship, everything has
the potential of being shared, so it is important for me to know what I
have brought to the table. I aim to suspend my thoughts and judgments
while being present and receptive to my patients.

I cannot over-emphasize the delicacy of sharing my embodied experience with my patients. For example, I could say that, "I am getting a
feeling of being torn apart or conflicted while working on your body."
In my experience, such words can be very powerful for patients, so I
say as little as possible. Very sensitive issues may arise. A number of
patients have admitted that they would not tell anyone else about the
feelings I have ventured to bring to the surface. Hence I am vigilant and
try to be as present, neutral and empathetic as possible.

Sometimes patients do not connect immediately with my embodied
experience revealed during the session, but will come back later with
some kind of meaning in response to my disclosure. There are also times
when my embodied response does not have meaning for my patients or
seems more meaningful to me. So I offer the experience and then take
an open approach to where it might lead. I am excited by the mystery
of therapy, by what a patient brings to the session as a whole person, by
what I am going to find, by what they going to find for themselves, and
by the open nature of where all this will lead to.

In conclusion, I have found the journey to becoming a MindBody
therapist is never-ending, but soulfully fulfilling. There is always
"something else."

References

Barral, J. P. (1996). *Manual thermal diagnosis*. Seattle, WA: Eastland Press.

Edwards, I. & Richardson, B. (2008). Clinical reasoning and population
health: Decision making for an emerging paradigm of health care. *Physiotherapy Theory and Practice, 24(3)*: 183–193.

Feldman, M. (2007). The illumination of history. *International Journal of
Psychoanalysis, 88(3)*: 609–625.

Finlay, L. (2006). The body's disclosure in phenomenological research. *Qualitative Research in Psychology, 3(1)*: 19–30.

Gallese, V. (2009). Mirror neurons, embodied simulation, and the neural basis of social identification. *Psychoanalytic Dialogues, 19(5)*: 519–536.

Gibson, B. E., Nixon, S. A. & Nicholls, D. A. (2010). Critical reflections on the physiotherapy profession in Canada. *Physiotherapy Canada. Physiothérapie Canada, 62(2)*: 98–100.

Grant, B. M. & Giddings, L. S. (2002). Making sense of methodologies: A paradigm framework for the novice researcher. *Contemporary Nurse: A Journal for the Australian Nursing Profession, 13(1)*: 10–28.

Nicholls, D. A. & Gibson, B. E. (2010). The body and physiotherapy. *Physiotherapy Theory and Practice, 26(8)*: 497–509.

Overmeer, T., Boersma, K., Main, C. J. & Linton, S. J. (2009). Do physical therapists change their beliefs, attitudes, knowledge, skills and behaviour after a biopsychosocially orientated university course? *Journal of Evaluation in Clinical Practice, 15(4)*: 724–732.

Ross, M. (2000). Body talk: Somatic countertransference. *Psychodynamic Counselling, 6(4)*: 451–467.

Sokolowski, R. (2000). *Introduction to phenomenology*. New York: Cambridge University Press.

Stone, M. (2006). The analyst's body as tuning fork: Embodied resonance in countertransference. *Journal of Analytical Psychology, 51(1)*: 109–124.

Soth, M. (2005). Embodied countertransference. In: N. Totton (Ed.), *New dimensions in body psychotherapy* (pp. 40–55). Maidenhead: Open University Press.

Upledger, J. E. & Vredevoogd, J. (1983). *Craniosacral therapy*. Seattle, WA: Eastland Press.

Wertz, F. J. (2005). Phenomenological research methods for counseling psychology. *Journal of Counseling Psychology, 52(2)*: 167–177.

CHAPTER TWELVE

Whakawhanaungatanga: establishing relationships

Iona Winter

Istood at the window of the *wharenui* (meeting house) and observed the darkened sky. A sudden storm was brewing. The trees began vigorously stretching their limbs, as birds skilfully rode the wind currents, engaging with the charged air. The roof above joined in, as the rain drummed its rhythm with increasing intensity. Water soon began its descent, spilling over the front of the *wharenui*, its breadth spread across the ground and to the stream beyond. Crashing thunder quickly unsettled me, as I waited for the flash which would follow. Everything, including me, was communicating and responding together, a natural radical integration.

This is a story of listening, seeing, feeling and sensing as a mind, body and spirit practitioner.

Ma te whakatau ka mohio, By discussion comes understanding,
Ma te mohio ka marama, By understanding comes light,
Ma te marama ka matau, By light comes wisdom,
Ma te matau ka ora. By wisdom comes life. (Robinson, 2005)

Timata—*Beginnings*

As a child I was keenly aware of the interconnectedness of everything around me. I was born and raised at the foot of the Waitakere Ranges, surrounded by bush, horse paddocks and orchards. We grew the majority of our fruit and vegetables, recycled everything, and rarely used the rubbish bin. My mother and I shared a gift of foreknowledge, and I would describe her as a spiritual person. She always seemed very in tune with her surroundings and would respond from a place of intuitive knowing. My father did not talk about having a spiritual belief system, but he taught me an appreciation of *Papatuanuku*, Mother Earth, the seasons and cycles of nature.

I can still recall as a child, during afternoon naps, the way the wind sounded through the curtain, the smell of the bush outside and the warm touches on my head by my *tupuna* (ancestors) as I drifted off to sleep. I sensed that I was part of something much bigger, "an interlocking universe" (Bowden, 2008). I grew up hearing, seeing, smelling and sensing *wairua* (spirit); it was present always and everywhere.

I often saw people in my room at night, and it was difficult to make sense of them. My mother chose not to see, despite her ability for foreknowledge, and would tell me there was not anyone there and that I should go to sleep. I knew there were people there, not real people with solid bodies, but people who were translucent. These people knew me and I had a sense of knowing them.

I loved exploring the *ngahere* (New Zealand forest), but because none of my girl friends were keen to "go bush" I would often tag along with my brother and his friends. Sooner or later, for a laugh, the boys would take off and leave me somewhere that felt really creepy. I would run to get out, often in blind panic, scared witless because the bush was full of *patupaiarehe* (fairies), who teased me relentlessly with their whispers, tickles and taunts.

There were however, at other times, magical moments by a stream where I would connect with a sense of timelessness and a feeling of deep inner peace.

School holidays were often spent with my maternal grandparents. My grandfather told us that the area they lived in had been a *pa* (Maori fortified village) site and I can still remember the feeling of profound sadness in the land there and how it seemed to move beneath my feet. There was an atmosphere of being watched by many unseen eyes, and as children we all felt it. This is how, as a child, I remember experiencing *te tapu o te whenua* (the spiritual element of land). I made sense of this through identifying with the *whenua* (land) and its previous inhabitants.

The physical realm is immersed and integrated with the spiritual realm (Pere, 1997).

My grandfather was a great teller of ghost stories. He had had many adventures in his life and would often talk with me about *te ao maori* (the world of Maori) and *te ao wairua* (the world of spirit). These talks contributed to the foundations and framework for my spiritual experiences. He saw *kehua* (ghosts) and this relieved me immensely; someone else could see what I was seeing.

As a teenager my sensing changed markedly. I saw much less than before, but dreaming, hearing and smelling became more acute. At age seventeen, my best friend was going away on holiday. Once we had said our goodbyes, I turned to the girl I was with and said, "I'm not going to see her again". A week or so later I dreamed that she had died. Upon waking that morning, I knew that she had gone and as the phone began to ring I knew it was her mother calling to tell me. I still wonder if she noticed my lack of surprise.

In my late teens I was devastated by the diagnosis of the early stages of cervical cancer. What followed was a journey of many recurrences and surgeries stretching into my mid-thirties. Frustrated by the lack of information and avenues for healing, I began to explore alternative therapies, which ultimately prevented the cancer from needing chemotherapy. I researched the stories of the women in my *whakapapa* (family tree), and a picture emerged of generations of abuse and trauma, most of which was unspoken and unresolved. I believe now that the cancers were a manifestation of this, and that it had come to me to work through and heal this cycle, to stop it passing on to the next generation.

Being a mother is the most amazing blessing I have known. I had never before felt so much connection to myself and my environment as I did when I was pregnant. It was as if all my senses were wide awake, I was seeing the world through a much clearer lens. Having been told that I had little chance of conceiving, because of my cancer history, this child was indeed a miracle. Tuning into him and his needs has been a powerful experience. As we learned to walk together, I was able to equip him with the skills and a language to articulate what he sees, hears and feels. My son is also *matakite* (a seer).

Whare Wananga—*University*

At age twenty six, after working as a counsellor for five years, I began university psychotherapy training and I struggled. My work until then had been about knowing and sensing, predominantly in an intuitive framework. I found I really did know things about the people I worked with, but was unable to rationalize how I knew them. Putting everything down to inherited knowing and intuition was unacceptable in the University. I needed to learn an academic and theoretical language, a language which did not really fit what I knew, a language that, at times, felt false. Curiously it was also a language in which I felt I was called upon to judge others. A radical integration was needed.

We are always in a state of knowing even when we do not realise it (O'Donohue, 1998).

During psychotherapy training the freedom of my knowing was greatly reduced. I did not listen to my intuition as much, and constantly questioned myself. My sense of *wairua* seemed to be partially disconnected, as if I was in limbo or missing a part of myself. I fought to be seen and heard, I clashed with tutors, and refused to diagnose cases on the basis of minimal information. I also rejected their interpretations of me, especially when they did not fit. I was labelled an angry adolescent, who would not conform to the dominant culture. Retrospectively, I acknowledge I was angry. I was angry that I was being asked to reject parts of myself, and I assumed they were not seen as valuable to my development as a therapist. Despite these challenges, I was determined to finish training as a psychotherapist. After seven years of juggling single parenting, part-time work and study, I did so.

Shortly after this, something happened to get me to tune in again to *wairua*. I received another positive cancer result and further surgery was advised. Part of me fought this. My body was tired, and I did not want more surgery. Through a friend, a Maori healer came my way and together we began to work on the abuse and trauma in my life, on a mind, body and spirit level. We worked on residues that had not been resolved through my previous psychotherapy. I was shown a path back to my knowing, listening, hearing, seeing and sensing.

I was invited to join *wananga* (a place of indigenous learning) and through this was introduced to *tohunga* (expert healer, mentor, priest) Hohepa Delamere; known to most as Papa. He taught me how to protect myself and my son, on a spiritual level. This learning built further on the foundations my grandfather had shown me. Papa suggested that perhaps I did not need the cancer anymore. Through a deep healing process the cancer I had battled for years went, because I was able to let it go. To say "letting go" may sound easy, but it was far from simple. The healing involved several years of intense body work, my own deep introspection, forgiveness, and learning to allow and trust men to assist me in letting go. I continued to heal and everything I had learned up to this point began to be integrated. It was clear that I had "recognition of interwoven causes within and around each person" (Bowden, 2010, p. 62).

In *wananga* I was with people who did not think it strange that I could sense things. Indeed the only thing my *wananga whanau* (family) thought was weird was why I would want to be a psychotherapist.

I started out on a new part of my journey, not only as a woman and mother but also now as a psychotherapist solidly connected to *wairua*. In my practice I became aware of the need to further consolidate and integrate my learning. There were times when I felt as though I was a fish out of water, floundering, unsure of how to rationalize the ways I worked. I will always be indebted to my supervisor, Lesley King. Through her skilful and generous participation in my growth as a therapist, we explored alternative languages for my style. As a result I gained more confidence as an emerging mind body spirit practitioner. It was through Lesley, some years later, that I heard about a new postgraduate university training programme in MindBody Healthcare, and I leapt at the opportunity. Here was a potential place of further learning, in the heart of academia. As I spoke my *mihi* (greeting) to the student group on that first day, I felt my *tupuna* standing beside me. It was extremely powerful and confirmed for me that I was in the right place.

One of the most important things for me during the training was learning new ways of articulating my practice as a Mind, Body and Spirit Psychotherapist. I found a sense of ease in speaking my truth, sharing my experiences and experimenting further with describing how I work; it was like a public radical integration. I had not, until this point, trusted that I would be able to do so without sounding like a circus fortune teller. I had been terrified of being seen as flaky. I am truly grateful for the acceptance, challenge and encouragement I received during this post-graduate training. I was stretched in many aspects of my being, and in ways I had never imagined.

Finding ways to normalize this integration in my daily work has taken time. Working in my own way, integrating my Maori/Celtic spirituality and healing framework with psychotherapy, my approach is now much more consolidated. I have continued to build upon my foundations and explored ways of working with my intuitions in a variety of settings.

Whakahangai—*Putting learning into practice*

For almost a decade, my employment as a counsellor and manager was at an educational institution located on land steeped in struggle, a battleground during periods both pre- and post- arrival of *Pakeha* (New Zealander of European descent) in Aotearoa, New Zealand. Later it became a psychiatric asylum.

Early on in my employment there it became obvious to me, due to the many disturbances staff and students intuitively felt, that our buildings were in need of *whakawatea* (clearing, blessing). This was something I was unable to do myself, given the size and history of the place, and so I contacted *kaumatua* (elders). It was important that, as a group, we blessed the building together with *kaumatua*, the result being that we talked often of the history. This assisted in raising the awareness of staff around *te tapu o te whenua*. One *kaumatua* likened *whakawatea* as "only wiping the surface". Too much had happened there, and unfortunately the *whenua* could never be fully cleared. We agreed that repeat blessings would be required each month, particularly given the work we did as counsellors and psychotherapists.

It was clear to me that a spiritual imprint remained, from all that had gone before. The numerous tragic deaths and battles had left a stain on the *whenua*. Interestingly, as I spoke about my feelings and experiences, other colleagues, who had mostly remained silent, began to talk. Over time I made many links between past events and present day experience for clients, colleagues and myself. It was important to me to maintain the spiritual health and well-being of the buildings we worked in.

I remember my first day there, walking into a building, like stepping through a portal into another time in which the air did not move. It felt thick with an almost palpable sadness.

The first experience of linking past to present, in this environment, was in working with a *Pakeha* client.

> My client was extremely angry, at the world, at men, and at herself. As she expressed her anger and linked her hands across her stomach, another face appeared out of her face and leered at me. It was like something from the science fiction film *Alien*. The face seemed to have surfaced from the depths, not only from my client but also the *whenua*. Soon after, the wall behind her head began to drip with green slime. I had experienced something like this before, but never in a client session. I remember shrieking internally, but knew I needed to stay calm and focused. Afterwards I was relieved to be able to debrief with Papa. I remember him laughing and saying, "Well, Bub, you are working in the old Maori psychiatric inpatient ward".

> For me this experience, while intangible, was nothing more, nor less, than what it seemed it was. Any attempt to make it conform to orthodox psychotherapy thinking seemed very likely to militate against being open to it. The sense I made of this experience was that "a monster" had surfaced from within my client. The conditions were ripe for its appearance; my client's ability to connect with her rage, my ability to witness the rage, and the shape it took, all being influenced by our surroundings.

> Traditionally for Maori (indigenous New Zealander) *te ao wairua* is a dimension which, for the most part, is unspoken for reasons of *tapu* or sacredness, but it is very present in everyday life. In more recent times, the importance of discussing traditional spirituality openly is being recognized. Thus Robinson calls for a new way forward: "where the old formula states that exposed knowledge becomes powerless, the new formula states that such knowledge remains powerful when people are able to receive its influence" (Robinson, 2005, p. 15).

Whakakotahi—*Integration*

Thus far I have attempted to show that my clinical practice is sustained by both deep experiential knowledge of the dimensions of mind, body and spirit, and trainings which include personal development within Maori culture and healing practices; as well as Western academic psychotherapy and MindBody training. I turn now to what happens in my office.

I see the therapeutic relationship and journey as a *waka* (vessel) for healing. My focus is on wellness rather than disease, and I am not diagnosis-centred. I sit with what is present, and endeavour to be with the client from my "undivided wholeness" (Bowden, 2008). I spend time before a first session tuning in, noticing my own mind, body and spirit. Sometimes I will notice any visitors (in spirit) present or messages from my own *tupuna* coming through.

The case example below illustrates how I may work with spirit.

> A Maori client I had was not listening to her *tupuna*. I knew this because they were trying hard to connect with her, and would often arrive before, during and after sessions and speak to me. I remember on one occasion the office door flew open, about fifteen minutes after she had arrived; it was as if she had forgotten there were some more visitors coming. She was angry that her *tupuna* had not protected her as a child. I would often hear the insistent *korero* (conversation) in my ears from a man who wanted to speak with her. Every time I mentioned this to her she would say: "What does he bloody well want?" or "I don't want to talk to him."

Shaw states that "Psychotherapy is an inherently embodied process" (Shaw, 2004, p. 271). Every so often I may get a pain in my chest, a headache or sore throat which comes on suddenly before, during or after a session. I do not necessarily read these as my own issues presenting in my body, but hold them with a tentative wondering as to whether these symptoms are mine, or a mirroring of my client's body state in some way. By using my body as a "tuning fork" (Stone, 2006) I have learned to listen (in a moment) to many things and trust my embodied listening.

Over the years I have found my most common somatic response is that I hold my breath. Strikingly, in my work with trauma, I feel much more in my body than I do with clients who do not sit in the trauma spectrum. Perhaps this is because I resonate on the same frequency, due to my own history. I agree with Orbach in that there is "no such thing as a body, there is only a body in relationship with another body" (2003, p. 10).

I strive to be holistic, interconnected, present, grounded, and aware of my body and breathing. By listening to, and reflecting upon, my counter-transferential thoughts, feelings and actions that occur during the non-verbal or somatic exchanges, clients are provided with a mirror for their somatic experiences.

I work with my *karaputaro*, my first thought, in its essence of knowing, simplicity and wisdom, as taught to me by Papa. *Karaputaro* differ from conclusions in that they come from a place of being fully present to all of me, the client I am working with, and the environment we are in.

Sometimes the work is focused upon supporting a person to find their own sense of wairua or spirituality in their lives. We draw strength from what they already know. I encourage clients to utilize their own resources, e.g. connections to nature, rather than imposing my own. "Through co-enactment—mutual perceiving—we give form" (Heron, 2006, p. 11). Spirit is an integral part of everything, and to separate it out would mean that my whole system would be out of balance. I see it as part of the whole, neither an exclusive more powerful component, nor non-existing.

While sessions with any client may often centre on emotions, I find ways to link them with their *tinana* (body), *te ha* (breath) and *wairua*. I enquire as to what my clients do for relaxation and exercise, and enquire as to their physical health and wellbeing. I may suggest a visit to a nearby Holistic Health Centre, or a visit to their general practitioner for a medical check-up.

If I am sitting with a client who is Maori, I explore what connection they have, or not, to their *whenua*. I often receive a very clear message. For example, they may need to go home and get their feet in their *awa* (river) or the *moana* (sea), or they may need to stand beneath a tree to connect with *Papatuanuku*. I find that simple things are often the most useful. Tuning in in this way enables me to find openings for enquiry with clients.

Ritual is involved in all my work, whether that is my own *takutaku* (ritual chant) before and after a session, or an inclusion of what my client may request from their spiritual frame of reference. Often this is a simple acknowledgement of the other with handshake, hug or hongi (noses pressed in greeting).

Taha Wairua—*The realm of spirit*

Occasionally I see clients' parents who have passed over, and if it feels appropriate, I might say something like: "Your Dad is right here beside you now, and he is really supportive in what you are doing" or "what do you think your Mum would say?" With Maori clients it is often easier because they usually have a clearer sense of their *tupuna* with them in their daily lives. I have also learned (over time) to carefully and sensitively translate what I hear the spirits saying, as it may not be politically correct or nice.

What follows is a case example of working in an integrated way with a Maori client.

> We had been exploring how sexual abuse had impacted on her relationships with men, and how she had an ongoing history of candida infection (thrush). Suddenly an old woman appeared at my client's right shoulder. She had a beautiful smile and was wearing an orange floral seventies style dressing gown. I took a breath and blinked to validate her appearance and she looked me straight in the eye and said:
>
> "I need you to pass something on to her. Tell her I am here to support her when she needs me. All she has to do is say my name and I'll be there".
>
> I intuitively felt this woman's appearance was timely to the topic of our session. Without question, her message needed to be passed on. By way of deduction, through my spiritual framework, I realized this must be my client's maternal grandmother.
>
> "Were you close to your grandmother?"
>
> "Oh yes, very close. She was so good to me when I was a kid. She had a very loud flowery dressing gown and I used to love snuggling up to her at night. She always looked after me. How come you ask?"
>
> "Well, she is standing behind you and has asked me to give you a message."
>
> "Oh my god, are you serious?"
>
> I told my client what I had seen and shared the message. Her eyes welled up with tears, overwhelmed that her grandmother had come to see us both, and especially at this time when she was feeling incredibly alone.
>
> After this session, my client began a regular dialogue with her Grandmother that she found very valuable. Her instances of candida were greatly reduced, and when we discussed this she put it down to feeling "much safer now Nan's back."

Spirits do not appear in a predictable fashion. I trust when they do appear that the timing is right, the channels of communication are open and a client is ready to hear their messages. This has however been a process of trial and error for me.

Aroha me te Aroaro—*Love and presence*

Most importantly, the therapeutic relationship is one of *aroha* (love). "In a climate of aroha, the psyche, the spirit of a person, can soar to great heights" (Pere, 1997, p. 6).

I am not a healer, my clients are, and our therapeutic relationship is a journey of shared healing; we both contribute to and gain from the process. By working consciously and with integrity, I am aware of clinical and relational safety and the need to hold my clients.

To be in the present, with all that is before and around me is important. If I have expectations of clients from an outcome focus, I am potentially interfering and limiting them from experiencing their own journey. By paying close attention to my breath, my body, sensations and movement, I move away from over-thinking. In connecting with myself, noticing without judgment and feeling the peace within, I am grounded.

"The moment you realise you are not present, you are present" (Tolle, 1999, p. 55).

I trust implicitly in my client's timing, respecting that when they are ready, the answers will come and the process of healing will take as long as it needs to. In letting go of time restraints and outcomes (perceived or projected) my clients are free to take their time.

As a practitioner it is necessary to acknowledge my *tupuna*, my guides and those who support me in the realm of *wairua*. Equally as important is appropriate supervision to balance my practice through reflection, wondering and questioning. In a modern Western context I work "outside of the square", but reassuringly a psychotherapy supervisor once said: "In working outside of the square, you are very aware of the square and your place in relation to it."

Kotahitanga—*Unity*

Safe practice is one which acknowledges and respects difference, and because of my nature it allows a place for *wairua* in every session. The "care of the soul is in many ways a return to early notions of what therapy is" (Moore, 1992, p. 5).

It amazes me what can lift my own spirits; a smile, a gesture, nature, a gentle hand on my shoulder, or the colours in the night sky. I do not underestimate the power of these things in my own life and within my *mahi* (work) with clients.

I acknowledge the interconnection of everything and everyone, regardless of culture.

"I am part of you and you are part of me, let us be in unity" (Delamere, 2002, personal communication).

My journey has indeed been one of radical integration. There are many things I came into this life already knowing through my *whakapapa*. Added to this is the learning from all who have loved, mentored, supported, challenged and encouraged me. I see my role as a facilitator for other healing journeys. A *tohunga* once told me that my gift is to hear and witness the stories of others. Ultimately, I would like to see developed an *Aotearoa* blend of psychotherapy, one which holds the values of *Tangata Whenua*, our indigenous people, and embraces the land on which I reside.

This wonderful path I am on will continue to be one of ongoing healing, coupled with the blessing of being mother to a wonderfully insightful son, and the challenge of continuing to work in the way that I do, combining Scottish, Irish, English and Maori world views. The radical integration lives in me, constantly ebbing and flowing with the seasons present in every day.

Kia tau te rangimarie, may you be in peace.

References

Bowden, R. (2008). *NZAP Conference*, Waitangi, NZ.

Bowden, R. (2010). Waka Oranga Hui-a-tau Presentation Notes. *NZAP Newsletter* (2010).

Delamere, H. (2002–4). *Personal wananga notes.*

Heron, J. (2006). *Participatory spirituality: a farewell to authoritarian religion.* Morrisville, NC: Lulu Press.

Moore, T. (1992). *Care of the soul.* New York: Harper Collins.

O'Donohue, J. (1998). *Eternal echoes.* London: Bantam Press.

Orbach, S. (2003). The John Bowlby Memorial Lecture-Part 1: There is no such thing as a body. *British Journal of Psychotherapy, 20(1):* 3–15.

Orbach, S. (2004). What can we learn from the therapist's body? *Attachment & Human Development, 6(2):* 141–150.

Pere, R. (1997). *Te Wheke. A celebration of infinite wisdom.* Gisborne, New Zealand: Ao Ako Global Learning New Zealand.

Robinson, S. T. (2005). *Tohunga.* Auckland, New Zealand: Reed Publishing.

Ryan, P. M. (2004). *The Reed pocket dictionary of modern Maori.* Auckland, New Zealand: Reed Publishing.

Shaw, R. (2004). The Embodied Psychotherapist: an exploration of the therapist's somatic phenomena within the therapeutic encounter. *Psychotherapy Research, 14(3)*: 271–288.

Stone, M. (2006). The analyst's body as tuning fork: embodied resonance in countertransference. *Journal of Analytical Psychology, 51(1)*: 109–124.

Tolle, E. (1999). *The power of now.* Novato, CA: New World Library.

http://www.maoridictionary.co.nz/index.cfm   date   last   accessed: 01/09/2012

CHAPTER THIRTEEN

Making a difference: a narrative MindBody approach to school guidance counselling

Yvonne Evans

Setting the scene

"Do you want to die or what?" These blunt words stopped me in my tracks. A teacher for over thirty years, a principal of a special school for fourteen years, working long hours with young people struggling to find their ways in life, I needed time to care for myself. Who was I, and what did I believe in? In hindsight, I had nearly lost myself. For example, in my rush, I had left the body of my dog with the veterinary surgeon, instead of bringing him home to be buried with the people he loved. He had been a faithful and loyal friend for fourteen years. It brings me pain to think about it even now. How did that happen? What was I thinking? At the very same time, the values and beliefs that had guided me as a teacher and school principal were being questioned by an educational system which, on the one hand, expected me to care for my staff and students, and address their health, safety and wellbeing, and, on the other hand, labelled my staff and me as "too" everything: "too caring, too understanding, too patient and too tolerant." I had naively assumed that government agencies were interested in and would do the right thing for youngsters without the knowledge, experiences, resources and power to do things for themselves. Shockingly, this turned out to be false.

For thirty one years I was a passionate teacher. I still am. I chose teaching as a vocation, guiding youngsters towards taking their place in our society, and then, in turn, trusting they would contribute to make all of our lives better. The education system is narrowly focused on the intellectual and physical aspects of personhood. Social, relational, environmental and emotional aspects of wellbeing are addressed through "key competencies", but they are not privileged in the way intellectual and physical aspects are. Spirituality is frequently ignored. Even when addressed, each aspect is attended to separately, especially in secondary schools with different teachers teaching different pieces of knowledge. This fragmentation of personhood is matched in its reduction-to-parts philosophy by the accepted view, in education, of people being individually responsible for their own lives. In New Zealand, recent trends of teaching to "unit standards" further mirrors this general pattern of fragmentation rather than holism. These ways of teaching are challenged by those who pursue alternative educational processes such as home schooling. There is less of a tendency to fragmentation in learning that is culturally-based such as *kura kaupapa* and bilingual units, where there is an emphasis on Maori language and ways of being, or in schools where religion is integrated into education.

Finding a way forward

I know the concept and reality of stress very well. I worked with young people (age five to fourteen years) facing illness or death in the family, family breakup, living in reconstituted families, relationship difficulties, physical health problems, and behavioural and learning difficulties. During a break from teaching, and working as a researcher, I investigated how teachers manage children's stress (Evans, 1996) and this led to a focus upon the importance of taking care of the whole person, the students and the teachers. On my return to school, my staff and I set about incorporating new activities, for both staff and students, to promote wellbeing; daily exercise, being connected, eating nutritious food, having opportunities to socialize, taking time to think and meditate, teaching young people problem-solving and peaceful ways of living, and external supervision for staff. Despite our best intentions and efforts, some of our staff members became physically sick. Something was missing.

While all this was going on, I noticed my body having a conversation of its own. In addition to high blood pressure, I developed rashes on my arms, shoulders and face. I experienced difficulty breathing, although I had never been asthmatic, and abscesses formed under my teeth. Bleeding from the bowel and strange, sore swellings in my abdomen led to several internal investigations. The medical conclusion, finally, was stress. When the school closed, most of the symptoms abated.

During my time as a researcher I had become aware of ideas from a narrative post-structuralist perspective, which opened a view of the world different from current school thinking and which later led me into pursuing a counselling career. My professional narrative counselling story has been configured by, firstly, a personal element, and, secondly, the whole person-oriented MindBody perspective.

Developing a narrative perspective

After the school shut down, I returned to university to complete my counselling thesis. I revisited the topic of stress, investigating how counsellors (and others in the helping professions) care for themselves and are cared for by others (Evans and Payne, 2008). From there, I became a guidance counsellor using narrative therapy, with its underpinning tenets of post-modernism and social constructionism informing my work. Knowledge, from a narrative post-structuralist perspective, emerges from one's personal and professional experiences, including professional training, and the meanings we make of them (Drewery, Winslade & Monk, 2000). Our shared humanity means we have much in common, but, in the end, personal knowledge and skills are structured around meanings derived from experiences filtered through values, beliefs, hopes and aspirations, which, because of the complexity of the human journey, appear as a highly idiosyncratic and individual story.

During my study, I was introduced to the importance of language and stories in living and wellness, becoming aware of discourses as dominant stories in our families and communities, and how these profoundly influence the decisions we make, the values we have, and the actions we take. I realized that the roles we play such as mother, daughter, student, teacher or friend are multi-storied. We are all members of communities and groups within our communities (defined by age, gender, socio-economic and cultural status, role in our family etc.). These memberships allow us to interpret life from unique viewpoints. The view that our lives are multi-storied allows us opportunities for choosing many different possible ways of being and living (Gergen, 1991), the very basis for narrative counselling. Personhood can be seen as arising from experiences in these roles (Davies & Harre, 1990). Through storying, we make meaning of events in our lives (Botella, Herrero, Pacheco & Corbella, 2004), by telling about and interpreting events in the dual landscapes of action and meaning (consciousness) in a way that creates coherence over the past, present and future (Bruner, 1990), and in a way that fits with how we think of life and the world (Gadamer, 1960). Through stories our identities are created, reviewed or changed (Angus, Lewin, Boufford & Rotoni-Trevison, 2004). Stories not only communicate ideas, they are a form of social action (Burr, 1997).

Problems can be viewed as arising from experiences that may not fit with the dominant discourse (Drewery, Winslade & Monk, 2000). In these days of globalization and cultural cross-pollination there is no one universal truth (Burr, 1997). Consequently, people are regarded as experts in their own lives, and having agency to make decisions and choose pathways, even if they need support at times to do so. Problems are not seen as deficits of the person (Bruner, 1990): "The problem is the problem, not the person is the problem" (Monk, Winslade, Crocket & Epston, 1997).

These new insights fitted well and extended the values, skills, and knowledge I had acquired helping youngsters as a special needs teacher. Whilst they now provided a satisfying basis for my work as a narrative counsellor, my personal view of holism and personhood was still dominated by the modernist, positivist, Western medical framework, and an education system which, because it typically separates out mind, body and spirit, meant that, as a school guidance counsellor, focusing upon the body was still off limits.

I had got so far, but, in the end, it was my own bodily illness response to my professional struggle that propelled me into exploring the MindBody connections by attending the New Zealand National MindBody Conference and then through post-graduate study in Mind-Body Healthcare at AUT University.

First light—gaining some knowledge and skills

Reading *The Body Speaks: Therapeutic Dialogues for Mind-Body Problems* (Griffith & Griffith, 1994) during a literature survey for my counselling thesis, further linked narrative to MindBody practice:

> … what to do when the expression of personal experience is not sufficient to resolve a symptom, because the personal narratives, or self-narratives, that are available to the patient hold the body in a symptom-producing bind. One must grapple with the destructive power of these stories—at times directly challenging their authority; at other times re-authoring old narratives, creating new narratives, or locating accessible but forgotten alternative narratives that do not engender symptoms. (Griffith & Griffith, 1994, p. 2)

However, incorporating MindBody concepts and skills into my narrative practice was immediately challenging. I had ethical concerns. How was a person previously not trained in working with the physical body meant to integrate the body into her practice? My own bodily perceptions had certainly changed for the better. I was much more aware of and appreciative of my own body, rather than treating it as a mode of transport for my mind. Here I was, a narrative counsellor, having to focus on the body. The MindBody studies certainly emphasized the power of words and stories, focussing upon "the patient's other story" (Broom, 1997), and, despite differences, this clearly overlapped with narrative therapy work. Exploring the importance of story-telling from an integrated mind, body and spirit perspective complemented my narrative ideas, confirming for me that storying is an essential human function: "We all need stories for our minds as much as we need food for our bodies … stories are motivating, rich in language experience and inexperience" (Wright, 1995). The next natural step seemed to be to develop an awareness of bodily and spiritual stories, bearing witness to them, making these stories more visible, and shifting the balance and focus to be more inclusive of mind, body and spirit in my professional work with youngsters. So began a journey of integration, of finding ways to honour the whole person; a journey that continues to this day.

The therapeutic value of stories is apparent in the *Dare to Move On* programme (based on the story *Smashed* (Hager, 2007)), which focuses upon young people getting into trouble through partying and abuse and eventually coming to the attention of the law. It skilfully explores issues such as identity, trust, peer pressure, abuse, drugs, sexuality, and consequences, giving rise to discussions on how to keep oneself safe and well. Using this programme with school groups, we encourage young peoples' own unique stories to emerge, hearing and honouring them; facilitating an emergent sense of emotional safety and integration. Discussions at this time come from a whole person perspective.

The MindBody framework of storying embraces the body. Linguistic metaphors were not new to me, but I had never considered diseases and illnesses as having meaning; even as somatic metaphors (Broom, 2002). The meaning of disease must be considered in the wider social, cultural, relational, spiritual and experiential sense, linking physicality and subjectivity, and individuality with community. Developing an awareness of the concept of somatic metaphor has invited me to examine and explore my thoughts about personhood, as well as offering me different positions from which to work with others, extending my narrative ways of working especially into the realms of body and physicality, previously unavailable because of the fracturing between mind and body. I have found a number of ways to bring mind and body into focus in the same time and space.

At one MindBody conference I encountered the Emotional Freedom Technique (EFT) which involves tapping certain parts of the body. EFT arose from meridian energy and thought field therapies, combined with ancient Eastern wisdoms, which consider that disease or illness occurs whenever there is a blockage or reversal of meridian energy within the body (Craig, 2011). Craig developed a method of tapping on various acupressure points to activate the energy flow while initiating thoughts and feelings which are then verbalized (Feinstein, 2008), and in the process enabling the body to return to a state of physical and emotional balance (Lambrou & Pratt, 2000). I quickly incorporated these skills into my own self-care and, after researching the science behind EFT during my MindBody studies, have found it useful for people to use in many situations including regaining calm, overcoming stress, and managing headaches and sleeplessness.

At another MindBody conference, Mindfulness and Focusing techniques caught my attention. Focusing developed within the humanistic school of therapies in the 1950s, specifically from the work of Eugene Gendlin and Carl Rogers. Contrary to what "experts" might hope for, clinical success was not so much determined by a therapist's qualities of "empathy, unconditional regard and congruence" (Hendricks, 2001) or "genuine caring, respect, acceptance and understanding" (Corey, 2001), but by the client's abilities to get in touch with feelings and inner self-knowledge. By encouraging clients to centre themselves, slow down and explore more thoroughly their "felt sense", Gendlin found people were often able to access new or different ideas about themselves. Crucially, from a MindBody perspective, this approach could be applied directly to bodily symptoms. "The felt sense is a sense of something before mind, body and spirit are split apart" (Hinterkopf, 2005, p. 215). By naming and accepting feelings in the throat, chest and abdomen areas, and then asking further questions, shifts in feelings and actions often resulted (Gendlin, 1981; Hendricks, 2001; Weiser Cornell, 1996). Integrating such ideas into my practice allowed new information to become available for people wanting to make changes in their lives. Mindfulness extends this idea, emphasizing the importance of just being in the present, providing the MindBody with rest from the stresses and strains of the modern world, and a chance to review what needs attention in our lives, as well as enabling presence with others and the forging of a healing partnership (Kabat-Zinn, 1999).

There was more to come. The focus so far had been upon the individual person, whether myself as therapist or my students. The fourth MindBody conference emphasized connectedness between and beyond individuals. Targ, in his book *Limitless Mind*, speaks of "the mind ... as unconfined by either space (brain or bodies) or time (present experience)" recognizing "that our nonlocal mind may effect healing both within and between people" (Targ, 2004, p. 143). In response, I found myself considering my own experiences and practices where connectedness may promote wellbeing. Personally, I had been on the receiving end of wonderful therapeutic connection; a feeling of being held in the hand, cared for, nurtured like a seed; enabling me to re-emerge from a world of darkness and despair, "to become" again.

As a teacher, the practice of connectedness had made a huge difference to my teaching. Schools are natural environments for connection, and students in despair may be drawn into activities with me such as breakfast club, peer mentor and peer mediation training, and wearable arts activities. They will be drawn in for many reasons, including wanting to help me out or merely by meeting other students who cross their path as they visit me, getting curious and then getting involved. This may then connect a distressed student with safe, interesting, caring people other than myself; allowing them to develop new friendships, trust and interests. Until recently, I had not appreciated how therapeutic these connections were in allowing distressed young people to move on in their lives to happier, more fulfilling places. At another level I am learning to use connection to inform my intuition as a basis for exploring new stories with people.

A new day—putting the MindBody approach to work

Guidance counselling in schools is a "one-stop shop" for young people who, mostly, have not as yet developed relationships with helping agencies. Until they come to secondary school, they are very reliant on the services provided (or not) by their families. In their quests for independence, young people tend to cut themselves off from previous help systems. Consequently, the guidance counselling job naturally becomes multi-facetted, fitting well with a MindBody approach. Conversations can range over many topics. Physical health and wellbeing conversations may visit eating and sleeping patterns, the management of stress and being sexually active, among other things. Mental, emotional and spiritual issues arise from social and relationship aspects of life. Conversations may explore thinking, problem solving, making sense of the world and making decisions, finding out who they are and how they want to live now and in the future, and how to communicate with significant others. Often our young people come from families struggling to live economically, socially and emotionally with insecure attachment patterns dominating their lives. I find myself discussing unwanted teenage pregnancies, disclosures of abuse and trauma, self-harm and suicidal ideation far too frequently. Many times it means finding a safe place for the young person to live as a start to addressing other issues.

This often means involving students with other professionals either inside or outside the school system; the drug and alcohol counsellor, public health nurse, doctors, Child and Adolescent Mental Health team, lawyers, police, court systems and social workers from other organizations such as Child, Youth and Family. Other adults within the wider family and friendship circles may need to be accessed for help. Despite accessing specialist help, my job as guidance counsellor is to coordinate the help, monitor progress and assist young people in building coherency in their narratives over the past, present and future that reflect their preferences.

Much of the work is self-referred and many other young people are referred by staff members, friends and family. Often this referral is part of addressing behavioural issues e. g., anger management, or lack of learning (school refusal, lack of attendance, and low levels of achievement); the primary concerns of schools. However, since staff are aware of my interest and willingness to explore the physical health care of students, they will now refer students with issues such as falling asleep in class or lacking their usual vitality, motivation and concentration.

My approach to conversations with young people is guided by a combination of narrative assumptions and a MindBody stance. Language and story are an integral part of both (Broom, 1997; White & Epston, 1990). Conversations usually begin with an invitation to speak about whatever is happening for them, allowing them to be the expert on their own lives (Monk, G.,Winslade, J., Crocket, K. & Epston, D., 1997) and to use the process for their own purposes with my listening from an open position (Broom, 1997) of curiosity or "not-knowing" (Monk, G.,Winslade, J., Crocket, K. & Epston D, 1997). At the same time I am becoming more attuned to the metaphors of the students' language (Broom, 1997; Kovecses, 2000) and the possibilities for meaning-making that arise from them. This is supported by a view of personhood as a coherent, integrated whole; a whole greater than just the sum of parts. Personally, I prefer to think of myself as "all things all the time"; my body as my mind and my mind as my body. Working with others from that perspective allows a wider range of stories and issues, including all aspects of wellbeing (physical, emotional, mental, spiritual, social and relational health) to be addressed than in my previous work. The ways of addressing the issues has changed as well, making use of a range of ways, like focusing, to access and use knowledge other than that produced cognitively and verbally. By placing an emphasis on attuned hearing and then using the specific language that the students use, I am able to develop a feel for the viewpoint from which they speak, as well as generating a perception of their being heard, understood and valued. In this way I become "decentred" (White, 1997), immersed in their world. I tend to start with the issues a young person finds most urgent and use my training and intuition to follow up on other issues until we have a more complete and coherent story.

On a daily basis I have found tapping, focusing, centering, meditation and focused bodily awareness useful in helping young people to manage uncomfortable and distressing feelings and bodily distress arising from events such as bullying, family illness, sleeplessness, lack of motivation and overwhelming anger.

> Jenny was a small girl for her age, both in stature and demeanour. She literally crept between classes at bell-time providing an invitation to less caring students to pick on her and have fun at her expense. She tried to remain unobtrusive at break times and always looked lonely, unhappy and scared. Whenever I approached her to ask if she was ok she said she was fine. I was sure she was being bullied and harassed. Eventually her father came to speak to me and Jenny agreed to see me when bullying events took place so we could confront the bullies. In addition, she agreed to see me every week in an effort to increase her own resilience. Working with her, I used centering, breathing exercises, and focusing; and Rothschild's (2003) idea of creating emotional anchors through associating thoughts and feelings with safe, happy events, times, places and people. Creating such connections is very useful in my practice to help young people and staff build resilience and wellness, feeling like they are in charge; especially when dealing with distressing or uncomfortable emotions, and in response to feelings of helplessness and powerlessness. I asked her to explore how her body was responding to the bullying. She identified the tension in her muscles, the faster, heavier beating of her heart, and her shallow, quicker breathing.
>
> In response to the questions, "Tell me about a time when you have felt very happy and had fun. Where was it and who was with you?"; she talked about a week she had spent at a Christian youth camp. We storied in detail the people, place and the events she enjoyed. I asked her to notice her body again. She smiled broadly; the first time I had ever seen her smile. She noticed that she was feeling more relaxed, her hands were warmer, her breathing more gentle. I asked what had happened and how she had done that. From that experience she came to understand and use a way of caring for herself in stressful situations; she would find a quiet spot and think about her time at camp. Working together over a period of eighteen months, Jenny became a happier, more settled student able to attend to her schoolwork.

I encounter many young people who self-mutilate or want to end their lives; both perhaps examples of profound disconnection. I help them to identify and story the feelings and events that have invited them into the situation. I ask them to identify where the emotional or physical pain is and explore where it came from. Focusing is often helpful in this process; accessing the body's own knowledge. Focusing can also provide some directions for dealing with the situation. My narrative therapy skills help me to deconstruct situations, identify and evaluate dominant discourses enabling people to reposition themselves in relation to the problem (Monk, G., Winslade, J., Crocket, K. & Epston, D., 1997; Morgan, 2000). New stories emerge based on their aspirations, hopes, values, and dreams which then evolve, leading to new beginnings and reconnection.

A number of other approaches have contributed to my MindBody ways of working. For example, Babette Rothschild's (2003) bodynamic running, running to a safe place, is another interesting way of working.

Marianna came to see me very upset because her closest friend, Nevis, had been removed from her home to live with her mother in the South Island. I asked her to story a journey from my room at school to Nevis' new home in the South Island. In response to my questions she described getting up from her seat, walking to the door, opening it and stepping out into our school grounds. In her mindbody, she ran down the path past the school buildings to the gate. When she got there she asked, "you are not going to make me walk all the way to the South Island are you, miss?"

With a giggle, I explained that a magic carpet was waiting there to fly her to Nevis. She happily climbed aboard and settled down for the ride. As she flew over the North Island she described the cities and physical features. Eventually we arrived in Dunedin.

"But I don't know where she lives miss, or what her house looks like."

"What did her house look like here? Will that do?"

She agreed we could use her old house as a template for our story. She stopped at the gate, walked up the path and knocked on the door. Nevis was so surprised to see her and threw her arms around Marianna saying, "What are you doing here?"

They went inside to talk. From then on Marianna knew she could be with Nevis whenever she wanted and her loneliness dissipated.

Another complementary technique is Michael White's "Re-membering conversations" (White, 1988) which I have found to be a powerful approach for fostering spiritual connections for bereaved students.

Ariana's parents had both been killed in an accident the year before I first met her at school. In that time, she had been removed from her siblings and the family home and brought to live with relations. After a few months with her extended family she was removed from their care because of an assault on her. In one year she had been in five different foster homes and had tried to kill herself six times.

A friend brought her to me in a distraught state. The first thing Ariana said was: "And I don't want to talk about my parents either!" I reassured her that I was only interested in talking to her about whatever she wanted to talk about. After doing some EFT tapping she calmed down enough to explain how lonely and disconnected she felt. She wanted to spend the weekend with her extended family, despite the previous abuse. We worked on that together for a couple of weeks and eventually she went back to live with her family with counselling support for all concerned.

However, before she left that first day I did invite her to come back and talk to me about her parents in the future if she wanted to. To my great surprise she turned up at my office the very next week. When I asked how she was and if there was something in particular she wanted to talk about, she said she wanted to talk about her Mum. We discussed what her Mum was like, what she did, what Ariana appreciated about her, and what Mum might say about the current situation. As we explored her beliefs about dying and death, Ariana explained that her Mum came and sat on the end of her bed every night. I wondered what she thought that was about. Ariana thought Mum knew she was distressed and was keeping an eye on her.

Over many months we had numerous conversations making Mum present by acknowledging Mum's thoughts, values and aspirations for Ariana. Mum was a member of her life in a different form now. The loss Ariana felt subsided. She settled down to living, learning, and became involved with peer mediation training so she could help others who had been through experiences like hers. She regained some purpose in life, resilience and happiness.

About eighteen months later she popped into my office for a chat. "Do you know Mum doesn't come and sit on my bed any more, miss?" We talked about what that might mean and she explained Mum knew she was okay now. Ariana was happy to let Mum be at peace too.

At times I actively explore spiritual beliefs with students especially after the death of a relative or when dying is imminent. Sometimes students raise questions about experiences they have of seeing people who have passed over, questions often prompted by a fear they may be insane; "it's not normal, miss." I usually ask them what beliefs they and their family have, whether these beliefs have been discussed and what they know; tuning into local insider knowledge (White, 2001). If asked, I share my own beliefs and experiences which seems to give them permission to speak about what may have been unspeakable up until that point (Griffith & Griffith, 1994).

Meeting a humourologist (a person who uses humour as therapy) at the first MindBody conference prompted me to read *Humor for Healing* (Harvey, 1998). This encouraged me to re-visit my own beliefs in the therapeutics of laughing and fun; something that has stood me in good stead throughout my life. I have reconnected with the ability to hold young people's attention, and the closeness of shared fun and laughter in the counselling rooms. I noticed that at times, after a particularly sorrowful or difficult session, students might go into the waiting room to recover before going back to class. Often a lot of laughter takes place at these times. What my reading did was explain that the students were busy releasing tension and balancing themselves; healing themselves one might say; ready to go back to class. Hearing Brian Broom speak (AUT lecture, 2006) about skin rashes from the perspective of human sensitivities that have been violated, of boundaries that have been crossed, and identities questioned, has had personal significance for me, as I have reflected on my past health issues. It also comes to mind when reflecting on some prolonged work I did with two young people with florid rashes.

Aaron, age fourteen, worked with me for two years until he left school. During the early stages he was in constant conflict with his peers. At least once a week he would be in my office with his friends or classmates sorting "stuff" out. Christine, age fifteen, worked with me for eighteen months addressing issues of school refusal, social isolation and living with a father who was perpetually drunk, keeping her up to the small hours of the morning on a regular basis.

After my work with them I noticed their rashes had gone. On reflection, I realized most of their issues related to teen identity; struggling to find out who they were, who they wanted to be, how to stand on their own two feet and have agency in their lives. Our work involved discussing their experiences and concerns, finding ways to realize who they wanted to be, how to grow up, and assisting them to achieve desired goals and grow their preferred reputations. I provided opportunity and information, emotional support and understanding in a safe environment, having conversations they did not have with other people. My MindBody work encouraged me to remain open to aspects of their bodily and spiritual experience, using these as metaphorical cues about what is going on for them.

This experience gives me food for thought about the acne troubles that teenagers struggle with at a time they are establishing their personal boundaries, designing their identities and futures, while feeling very sensitive to criticism. My work with Zara illustrates the multifaceted issues that typically arise in my workplace on a daily basis:

Zara was an interesting student I had initially met in year nine. Although she was very capable, she was not achieving; she seemed distracted by the task of growing up and becoming independent. Zara was popular with her peers. At times she was capable of being a strong leader, and at other times a follower. She had strength of character I admired, being fiercely loyal and supportive of her friends. Although her father seemed the stronger of her parents, he was in a new relationship and had had suicidal feelings which the extended family blamed on Zara's behaviour. From Zara's point of view, her father's new relationship had left Zara feeling put aside: "He no longer has any time for me, miss." She also reported: "Mum has been on happy pills."

Zara tended to turn up at my office in times of crisis; such as when her grandfather with whom she was really close died, her parents split up, she became pregnant, had a termination, and then split up with her boyfriend. Although she was physically fit and an active sportsperson, she smoked, drank, and used drugs recreationally. Twice she turned up at the counselling rooms saying, "I keep wanting to cry but I don't know what for." When exploring this she saw no connection between the challenges and changes she was facing in her life and her feelings. She had been referred to Child and Adolescent Mental Health Service by her family without any improvement in her wellbeing. After a week on stress leave from school, she agreed we needed a different plan of attack to her spasmodic attendance at counselling in times of crisis.

One of Zara's less endearing qualities was her brash, abrupt way of speaking. This meant that she was not very well liked by some staff, who saw her as rude, self-opinionated and uncooperative. My years of working with students with socially, emotionally and educationally demanding behaviours allowed me to see past these qualities and appreciate Zara from a different point of view; her intelligence, sense of justice, her loyalty to her own beliefs and friends, and her openness. I admired the honesty with which she communicated to me. My skill of putting things aside and paying attention to other qualities fitted well with both my narrative way of working (Madsen, 1999) and my MindBody approach (Broom, 1997). In doing so we were able to have discussions about some of her qualities, hopes and dreams for her future life and identity. My knowing different things about her helped to keep us connected and engaged. My acceptance of her allowed her to visit whenever she needed.

At one stage we had a discussion about being sexually active and what was in this for her; what did she get out of the experience? This approach to teenage sexuality, in contrast to the futility of asking why young people take the risks they take, arose from work by Tolman (2002). After an exclamation of, "Exactly, miss!" the question gave rise to an interesting discussion of the discourses surrounding being sexually active as a young woman; doing things to please others rather than yourself, giving in to peer pressure, living with the possibility of a reputation you do not like, and exploring the differences the community expectations have for young women and men. The discussion concluded with a shift in attitude towards considering being sexually active in her own time, and as part of the overall plan of life rather than a random experience.

What the new day looks like

Building on my own experiences as well as having opportunities for robust conversation, study, and supervised clinical practice have allowed me to shift my focus in practice to a more integrated approach. This shift has enabled me to take better care of myself and assist others. Using a narrative approach, multiple stories of young people's lives are honoured and made available to be used as a valuable basis for change. Intuition has been legitimized to inform practice. Professional boundaries have become clearer, addressing my own need for clarity around ethics. New skills have added to a growing confidence in my own practice, providing courage to try new things. All in all, new knowledge has provided more options for making a difference. However, apart from conferences, appropriate and affordable professional development is difficult to access. Another challenge arises from my geographical isolation from other MindBody practitioners in large centres meaning that regular, appropriate clinical supervision is not available to further stretch and stimulate my practice.

Changing to an integrated MindBody narrative form of practice has had the strange outcome of making me more connected to some professionals, and more isolated from others. Working with people who think and practice in an integrated way is tremendously exciting, almost all-consuming in the innovations and changes required; something like slowly opening a door to a vast new room. At the same time I find myself disconnected from many professionals who think and practice within the traditional Western biomedical model, the body-only orientation, which Dossey calls Era 1 medicine (Targ, 2004). Not only has this meant changing my own doctor, but in my workplace I have to be cautious with other health professionals with whom I work. They do not expect me to have knowledge about or attend to physical wellbeing. Some resent my intrusion into their field of expertise. Teaching staff and parents sometimes question my having conversations about integrated wellness. It is comforting at these times to have a university qualification in MindBody Healthcare.

What the future holds…

Reflecting on my MindBody journey thus far invites a question of how long this journey might take, and where it might lead. Probably the rest of my life, to who knows where? Saki Santorelli (1999) echoes these ideas when he says,

> Just like you, I remain a student, continually finding my way. I am bewildered and endlessly amazed by the mindlessness I encounter in myself, awed by the genius before me in the likeness of those who seek my care and give me so much, and grateful for the countless opportunities to practice wakefulness within the community of my colleagues and those whom I meet… in this vast, edgeless domain. (p. 3)

In which case, I am assured the path will be exciting, challenging and life-changing both for the people with whom I work, and for me.

References

Angus, L.E., Lewin, J., Boufford, B. & Rotoni-Trevison, D. (2004). "What's the story?" Working with narrative in experiential psychotherapy. In: L. E. Angus & J. McLeod (Eds.), *The handbook of narrative and psychotherapy: Practice, theory and research* (pp. 87–102). Thousand Oaks, CA: Sage.

Botella, L., Herreo, O., Pacheco, M. & Corbella, S. (2004). Working with narrative in psychotherapy: A relational constructivist approach. In: L. E. Angus and J. McLeod (Eds.), *The handbook of narrative and psychotherapy: Practice, theory and research* (pp. 119–136) Thousand Oaks, CA: Sage.

Broom, B. (1997). *Somatic illness and the patient's other story: A practical integrative mind/body approach to disease for doctors and psychotherapists.* London: Free Association Books.

Broom, B. (2002). Somatic metaphor: A clinical phenomenon pointing to a new model of disease, personhood and physical reality. *Advances, 18 (1):* 16–29.

Bruner, J. (1990). *Acts of meaning.* Cambridge, MA: Harvard University Press.

Burr, V. (1997). *An introduction to social constructionism.* New York: Routledge.

Corey, G. (2001). *Theory and practice of counseling and psychotherapy.* Belmont, CA: Brooks/Cole.

Craig, G. (2011). *EFT (Emotional Freedom Techniques) the EFT manual.* Santa Rosa, CA: Energy Publishing Press.

Davies, B. & Harre, R., Positioning: The discursive production of selves. *Journal for the Therapy of Social Behaviour, 20 (1)*: 43–63.

Drewery, W., Winslade, J. & Monk, G. (2000). Resisting the dominating story: Toward a deeper understanding of narrative therapy. In: R. A. Neimeyer & J. D. Raskin (Eds.) *Constructions of disorder,* pp. 243–263. Washington, DC: APA.

Evans, Y. (1996). *How teachers handle children's distress.* (Report prepared for the Ministry of Education Research Affiliate scheme). Hamilton, New Zealand: University of Waikato, Department of Education Studies.

Evans, Y. & Payne, M. (2008). Support and self-care: professional reflections of six New Zealand school counsellors. *British Journal of Counselling, 36 (3)*: 317–330.

Feinstein, D. (2008). Energy psychology: A review of the preliminary evidence. *Psychotherapy: Theory, Research, Practice, Training. 45(2):*199–213.

Gadamer, H. G. (1960). *Truth and method.* New York: Seabury.

Gendlin, E. T. (1981). *Focusing.* New York: Bantam Books.

Gergen, K. J. (1991). *The saturated self: Dilemmas of identity in modern life.* New York: Basic Books.

Griffith, J.L. & Griffith, M. E. (1994). *The body speaks: Therapeutic dialogues for mind-body problems.* New York: Basic Books.

Hager, M. (2007). *Smashed.* Auckland: Random House.

Harvey, L.C. (1998). *Humor for healing: A therapeutic approach.* San Antonio, Texas: Therapy Skill Builders.

Hendricks, M. N. (2001). Focusing-oriented/experiential psychotherapy. In: D. Cain & J. Seeman (Eds.), *Humanistic psychotherapy: Handbook of research and practice* (pp. 221–252). Washington, DC: American Psychological Association.

Hinterkopf, E. (2005). The experiential focusing approach. In: L. Sperry & E. P. Shafranske (Eds.) *Spiritually oriented psychotherapy* (pp. 207–234). Washington, DC: American Psychological Association.

Kabat-Zinn, J. (1999). Foreword in S. Santorelli, *Heal thy self: Lessons on mindfulness in medicine.* New York: Three Rivers.

Kovecses, Z. (2000). *Metaphor and emotion: Language, culture, and body in human feeling.* Cambridge: Cambridge University Press.

Lambrou, P. & Pratt, G. (2000). *Instant emotional healing: Acupressure for the emotions.* New York: Harper-Collins.

Madsen, W. (1999). *Collaborative therapy with multi-stressed families: From old problems to new futures.* New York: Guilford Press.

Monk, G., Winslade, J., Crocket, K. & Epston, D. (Eds.). (1997). *Narrative therapy in practice: The archaeology of hope.* San Francisco: Jossey Bass.

Morgan, A. (2000). *What is narrative therapy? An easy-to-read introduction.* Adelaide: Dulwich Centre Publications.

Rothschild, B. (2003). *The body remembers casebook: Unifying methods and models in the treatment of trauma and PTSD.* New York: W.W. Norton.

Santorelli, S. (1999). *Heal thy self: lessons on mindfulness in medicine.* New York: Three Rivers.

Targ, R. (2004). *Limitless mind: A guide to remote viewing and transformation of consciousness.* Novato, CA: New World Library.

Tolman, D. L. (2002). *Dilemmas of desire: Teenage girls talk about sexuality.* Cambridge, MA: Harvard University Press.

Weiser Cornell, A. (1996). *The power of focusing: A practical guide to emotional self-healing.* Oakland, CA: New Harbinger Publications.

White, M. (1988). Saying hullo again: The incorporation of the lost relationship in the resolution of grief. *Dulwich Centre Newsletter, 3*: 14–21.

White, M. (1997). *Narratives of therapists' lives.* Adelaide: Dulwich Centre Publications.

White, M. & Epston, D. (1990). *Narrative means to therapeutic ends.* New York: Norton.

Wright, A. (1995). *Storytelling with children.* Oxford: Oxford University Press.

CHAPTER FOURTEEN

Becoming an intimate lecturer

Marlies Dorrestein

Introduction

I have explored MindBody philosophy for many years, mostly as a personal journey. Recently I have begun to actively and deliberately integrate this philosophy into my work. I share this deeply internal and personal story because I think it has relevance and value in relation to an aspect of occupational therapy and occupational therapy education that is insufficiently recognised and addressed, namely the influence of the internal experience of the therapist or educator on the relationship with clients or students.

My personal health story

In January 2003 I found myself splattered against a wall after learning that the tumour that had been removed from my abdomen was malignant. My experience of the healthcare system as a patient was mixed; the high levels of professional and technical skill demonstrated by my health care providers stood in stark contrast to how irrelevant I felt as the person in that situation. The health professionals treated my tumour and my body as a physical entity that needed to be fixed, instead of approaching my current health situation in a collaborative way and in the context of my life as a person. The sense of depersonalization was captured for me in being seen and labelled as a patient, rather than as a person.

The medical team decided that chemotherapy and radiation therapy were not necessary and the surgeon told me that I could now "put it all behind me." This recommendation did not reassure or satisfy me. The Internet provided information about the forty percent of people who died within five years but nothing about what the other sixty percent were doing to survive. I went into a retreat centre for a week-end to gather myself, and found information about cancer and whole-person cancer approaches that made sense to me and gave me hope. The Cancer Foundation of New Zealand informed me that they did not provide information about whole-person approaches to dealing with cancer, since no one approach had been proven effective. Yet I had a strong sense and belief, that if my internal and external environment had generated this tumour, then I needed to change this environment in order to minimize the chances of the cancer recurring. My healthcare practitioners variously dismissed, ignored, or somewhat patronizingly acknowledged my views. Much later I came across research that sup-ported my belief (Cunningham & Watson, 2004). Additionally, having been through a long and slow process of uncovering, integrating and healing some emotionally and spiritually challenging family history, I understood the tumour to have a symbolic meaning in relation to my life experience. I later found supporting evidence for this radical notion in a medical context when I read Broom's books (1997, 2007) during MindBody postgraduate study started in 2010.

A few months after the surgery I participated in a programme called "Creative Healing"®, co-created by nurse and psychotherapist Bev Silvester-Clark (n.d.), that had an intentionally integrative mindbody and spirit healing focus (Stanfield, 2003). The programme translated scientific evidence and traditions of knowledge (for instance Booth, 2001; Kabat-Zinn, 1996; Myss & Shealy, 1999; Pert, Dreher & Ruff, 1998) into practical applications to facilitate healing. Applying these practical applications in my life, I recognized a strong relevance to occupational therapy's foundational principles, but saw limited acknowledgement of these links within occupational therapy practice. Some examples from my own experience are: the intrinsic impact of what I do and par-ticularly how I do it on my health (i.e., meaningful occupation does not necessarily translate into improved health), the effect of meditation on my well-being (i.e., not-doing and developing a heightened awareness of and changing how I do in my life), and the importance of a facilitating (or therapeutic) relationship in influencing my process of moving into more healthful living. The programme built on my longstanding personal interest in spiritual and emotional development and healing, and sparked my interest in a MindBody approach to health care. I felt frustrated and disillusioned at the apparently complete absence of support for, or even interest in, this kind of approach within the conventional health context, in spite of the significant benefits that had been demonstrated (Stanfield, 2003) and that I had experienced. I yearned for a greater degree of integration between my personal beliefs and experiences, and my chosen health care practice.

In 2008 I accepted a position as university lecturer in occupational therapy, after thirty years as a practitioner. One of several intentions was finding a way to incorporate an evidence-based approach to the above interests into my work and occupational therapy practice in general. I enrolled in the Masters in Health Science (MindBody Healthcare) a couple of years later. What follows is my story of how I have started to integrate a MindBody approach into my teaching role, with some indications of the link to occupational therapy practice.

Trying to find a fit in education

My transition from practising occupational therapy to teaching it in a tertiary health education context was exciting, full of potential and initially deeply challenging. One of my reasons for moving into education was that I had had positive educational experiences and feedback during my work in residential care for older persons, with care staff, activity staff and occupational therapy students. However, my sense of having something to offer as a person quickly diminished once I started working as a lecturer. I found myself in a strongly cognitive and Western scientific academic domain, with pressures around deadlines, research outputs, impact factors, large cohorts of students, curriculum content, assessment, fast pace, high workloads, and "doing, doing, doing"(personal journal entry, October, 2010). I could not imagine myself further away from a health-promoting MindBody context, in spite of occupational therapy's return to the holistic core construct of occupation and the significance of the meaning of occupation (Reed,

Hocking & Smythe, 2010), and to spirituality being acknowledged as being in the centre of one of the main models of practice; client-centred practice (Parker, 2006; Townsend & Polatajko, 2007).

Participating in professional development on tertiary teaching, I learnt some useful teaching techniques and theory. Yet I questioned why I had thought I would enjoy teaching, as I did not feel resourced to address some of the issues I was experiencing. For example, when teaching large groups of students, up to one hundred in a lecture theatre, all I could see from the lectern was a sea of blank faces. I struggled with making connections with the group, and at times I felt angry at what I saw as the students' lack of commitment, lack of respect, lack of interest, and lack of involvement in what I had so conscientiously organized for their benefit. The external and departmental supervision I received during the first couple of years mostly assisted me not to take the struggles too personally, as senior colleagues indicated that they also still struggled in a class at times. In spite of all of this I had a sense that in this work environment I would find a way to fulfil some of my aspirations.

Studying the MindBody Healthcare papers began to reveal the potential to bring at least some of my personal and professional domains together. To start with, I endeavoured to articulate the subtle differences between occupational therapy and MindBody healthcare perspectives on the concepts of holistic practice and client-centred-ness. In occupational therapy literature, holistic practice is described as encompassing a more inclusive perspective than many other professions in the Western healthcare system. As an occupational therapist I recognize a person as a complex whole being, "attending to emotional, cognitive, social, and physical aspects rather than homing in on isolated parts" (Finlay, 2001, p. 269). I draw on a variety of conceptual practice models "in order to achieve a comprehensive understanding of a client from multiple perspectives" (Kielhofner, 2009, p. 283). Additionally I am aware of the interdependence of person, environment and occupation (Townsend & Polatajko, 2007) and work "towards the simultaneous health of all parts, ... body, mind, emotion, and spirit" (Hemphill-Pearson & Hunter, 1997, p. 37).

When exploring holism from a MindBody perspective, I found the focus shifting subtly to a fundamentally different domain. In this domain the physical, subjective, social, sexual, cultural, behavioural and spiritual are not seen as separate parts, but as an essentially inseparable (i.e., non-dual) multi-dimensionality of a whole person.

These multiple dimensions arise at the same time as expressions or manifestations of each other, which co-create a person's health status or condition (Broom, 1997). In addition, along with my own experience, Lipton (2005), Wisneski and Anderson (2005) and Broom (1997, 2007) found that the importance and meaning of our own personal life experiences have a significant effect on a person's immune function and health or disease. Finally, I learnt that in a non-dual MindBody holistic approach the personhood of both the health practitioner and the person seeking assistance for their health condition are intimately and mutually influential on each other (Siegel, 2010; Svenaeus, 2000).

Translating some of the above into an education context, I was grappling with being a lecturer, a therapist, a postgraduate student and a person. It felt as if these roles existed as separate parts of my being and demanded separate behaviour and a separate language in different contexts at different times. I was concerned with finding a way to bring my current roles as educator and occupational therapist into a whole person-centred MindBody framework.

I saw that there was one way to bring these roles together. In the first instance I needed to be myself as a person and find a way to teach the students the importance of being a person who is willing to walk alongside another person, listen for what may be at the core of his or her concerns and respond to him or her in a place of heart-felt human connectedness and openness. This seemed to be a crucial element of client-centred, or rather whole-person-centred practice. All of the other's meaningful life experience needs to be seen, welcomed and acknowledged in the interpersonal encounter, as a foundation for using all occupational therapy knowledge and skills.

I would have experienced a very different healthcare journey in 2003, had more of my own health providers embraced this approach. I found only two authors in the occupational therapy literature who addressed this specific perspective. Johnson (1996) and Bridle (1999) identified and provided examples of the need to listen for the emotional meaning in a person's health story in order to enhance the occupational therapy intervention. In addition, Johnson (1996) specifically stressed the importance of creating a therapeutic relationship which incorporates intimacy and authenticity, i.e., dealing with our own feelings and emotions in order to have the capacity to address a person's emotional pain and sadness, and the importance of "address(ing) the mind-body relationship" (p. 395). Based on all these insights, I wanted to incorporate the information gained from my own lived experience and internal world into the therapeutic encounter, in my case the educational encounter.

I was beginning to see that in education, as in MindBody healthcare, the relationship with another person and awareness of our own multi-dimensional selfhood were probably paramount. At that stage I had not started exploring the evidence for this notion in education, and I had not arrived at how I might be able to bring this understanding into practice. My wonderings about this were confirmed later on in my reading of Palmer's (2007) seminal work on transformative education and several other books and articles since then, including some within the occupational therapy literature (Peloquin, 2002; Wood, 2004).

Intimacy, lived body and mindfulness

Spurred on by the memory of my own healthcare experience and inspired by what we were learning about the therapeutic relationship within an integrative MindBody healthcare framework, I started exploring the concepts of intimacy, lived body and mindfulness. While they appear to be quite different and separate concepts, the sections that follow demonstrate how I experienced them as intimately interlinked.

Intimacy

"Intimacy" and "relationship" are fundamental elements in the Mind-Body healthcare process, so I began to explore them within my personal and professional life. Learning to work within a framework that recognizes the multi-dimensional nature of individuals and their relationships is complex. I found support in literature on the therapeutic relationship, i.e., the intimate interpersonal space between health practitioner and person, and learnt that it needs to be carefully negotiated and held, in addition to appropriately facilitating the person's need to stay in control (Astin, Shapiro, Lee & Shapiro, 1999). I knew from my own life and professional practice in working with older people with dementia, building a therapeutic relationship and using intimacy skills is essential when engaging the person in the healthcare process. This engagement is recognized as an important factor in achieving positive health outcomes (Cole & McLean, 2003; Gruman, J. Rovner, M. H., French, M. E., Jeffress, D., Sofaer, S., Shaller, D. & Prager, D. J. 2010; Roter, Stashefsky-Margalit & Rudd, 2001), both in mainstream and (even more so) in MindBody healthcare.

In bringing more awareness to my own way of being, I saw intimacy everywhere, with clients, in my own therapy, in the work environment, with friends, and in meeting new people. I experienced the need to manage and balance the deeply human need for connection and belonging, with the need to maintain personal and professional safety. I was able to do that in dementia care; the other person posed no threat to me, and I found it easy to honour the totality of the person they are and have been. I realized that in endeavouring to model deeper interpersonal skills within the more threatening academic context, I would be confronting my own relational issues, in interacting with academic colleagues and with groups of students e.g., in lectures and tutorials.

I started to take note of the degree to which I was living relational qualities such as kindness, warmth, openness and compassion in my daily interactions with colleagues and students. This was a sobering process. It highlighted emotional intimacy as a dimension that is not only challenging in a personal context, but even more so in a work context. I was aware of the fear of not measuring up to perceived academic expectations and fear of the power of groups of students. I noticed my return to habitual patterns of behaviour on several occasions, such as wanting to hide within my professional role or the return of a lack of confidence about my role as an educator. I realized that if I wanted to instil the importance of intimacy in the therapeutic relationship, and impart skills of compassionate practice within a healthcare context, I had to find a way to model these skills, live this way of being, both with my colleagues and the students, and learn to articulate this knowledge in a way that is valid within an academic context.

Lived body

As part of the Mindbody Healthcare Master's programme, I explored knowledge and insights on the nature of body from an integrative MindBody perspective. This created a sense that my own body provides the most fundamental way through which I experience my personhood, and my lived body is the place through which my experience finds meaning and (eventually) language to express that meaning (see for example, Toombs, 1988). Even though occupational therapy knows or affirms the importance of the lived body and the embodied mind (Kielhofner, Tham, Baz & Hutson, 2002), I recognized a new level of experiential knowing. It felt like a revelation.

It took me several months to discover what was new in this realization; that I can utilize body-focused awareness to inform my responses on a moment-by-moment basis. Over the previous twenty years I had been gradually getting more in touch with the felt sense of my body. In contrast, I had often expressed my sense of the much greater importance of my internal/thinking/feeling/emotional world over my external/physical world. At the same time I was aware that a lot of this internal world did evidence itself through my body, even to the extent of producing an abdominal tumour, which I understood without doubt to be a somatic metaphor. However, I could not see at that time how I could and would make practical use of my newly gained awareness. I decided to engage in some body-work. As a result of the body-work, the ongoing study, and body-centred psychotherapy and supervision, I started to feel more present and connected with my body, more often able to stay in open and intimate relationship and connect from a solid centre in communication with students and colleagues.

Mindfulness

A colleague's presentation about how her meditation practice was influencing her teaching inspired me. I recognized the potential for including mindfulness in my teaching practice in the context of a Mind-Body framework and in the context of my drive to bring several threads of my personal and professional interest and development together. I have had a personal interest in meditation for many years, and have experienced the benefits of it for my own health and well-being, but it had not occurred to me to consciously bring mindfulness practice into my role as an educator. I recalled that a mindful way of being consists of attitudinal qualities of non-judging, patience, gentleness, generosity, empathy, gratitude (Kabat-Zinn, 1996), as well as acceptance, openness, and curiosity (Siegel, 2007). Additionally, Brown, Ryan and Creswell (2007) described evidence that regular mindfulness practice enhances our ability to be present in the world and in our relationships.

Searching the literature I found that meditation, described by Yuasa as "a mediating (process) between mind and body" (cited in Nagatomo, 1992, p. 71), has a comfortable fit with MindBody practice. Meditation allows access to the unconscious and the personal experience of the non-dual nature of our MindBody (Kabat-Zinn, 2011). This occurs through noticing, observing and assessing all of our multi-dimensionality with a non-judgmental attitude (Kabat-Zinn, 1996). Nagatomo (1992) includes in this our thoughts and images, while the breath, sensory responses within our physical body, and feelings, are dimensions identified by Kabat-Zinn (1996). As a result of attention to all these dimensions, meditative practice allows deeper insights than those able to be accessed through rational thinking (Zajonc, 2009), and provides a non-conceptual understanding (Grabovac, Lau & Willett, 2011), and changes in the MindBody "physiological coherence" (Hart, 2004, p. 31). These were processes that I had witnessed and experienced.

Additionally, I found evidence that mindfulness-based approaches are now well accepted in healthcare as MindBody interventions that improve physical and psychological wellbeing (Grossman, P., Kappos, L., Gensicke, H., D'Souza, M., Mohr, D. C., Penner, I. K. & Steiner, C. 2010; Hede, 2010). I knew that mindfulness approaches are comprehensively discussed within psychotherapy and counselling (see for example Didonna, 2009; Hick & Bien, 2008). I discovered that discussion on mindfulness is starting to emerge in occupational therapy (Hawtin & Sullivan, 2011; Thompson, 2009). Gockel (2010), Irving, Dobkin, and Park (2009), Stew (2011), and others describe benefits of mindfulness in the education of student health professionals. Additionally mindfulness has been demonstrated as a successful stress management approach for health professionals and educators (Anderson, Levinson, Barker & Kiewra, 1999; Christopher, J. C., Chrisman, J. A., Trotter-Mathison, M. J., Schure, M. B., Dahlen, P. & Christopher, S. B. 2011; Hede, 2010; Irving et al., 2009).

I am most familiar with mindfulness as an integral part of a Buddhist philosophical, spiritual, and mind-training approach, because I was introduced to it and had practised in this context, since the early 1990s. There is a lot of variety in how mindfulness is understood, even within Buddhist traditions and history (Gethin, 2011; Kang & Whittingham, 2010). I include some of the descriptions I have found helpful and have applied in the context of my journey of MindBody practice integration. From a Buddhist perspective mindfulness has been described as: "bare attention, … the clear and single-minded awareness of what actually happens *to* us and *in* us, at the successive moments of perception" (Thera, 1996, p. 30, original emphases), "keeping one's consciousness alive to the present reality" (Nhat Hanh, 1975, p. 11), and "to see clearly and directly the truth of our experience in each moment" (Goldstein & Kornfield, 1987, p. 5).

I found it useful to make the distinction between "formal" and "informal" mindfulness meditation practice. Formal mindfulness practice is described as "specific periods of time in which we purposefully stop other activity and engage in particular methods of cultivating mindfulness and concentration" (Kabat-Zinn, 2005, p. xx). Informal mindfulness practice can be identified as the endeavour to bring a mindful state of being and qualities of mindfulness to our everyday activities, interactions and being in the world (Kabat-Zinn, 2005; Nhat Hanh, 1975/1987). While I do not always manage to engage in a daily formal meditation practice, this did not stop me from integrating informal mindfulness into my teaching practice.

Mindfulness as a MindBody approach in education

Once I started searching for relevant literature on mindfulness in education, I discovered that education, including tertiary education, has also embraced the spiritual domain and contemplative practice (Palmer, 1993, 2007; Palmer, Zajonc, Scribner & Nepo, 2010; Zajonc, 2009) in its curricula, because of proven benefit in a variety of domains that are valued within an educational context (Hart, 2004). I found that the main focus in the literature on contemplative education is the improvement of students' cognitive and academic performance, and positive effects on students' mental health and well-being. Additionally benefits have been identified for the development of the whole person (Miller, 2006), specifically in interpersonal relationship functioning (Shapiro, Brown & Astin, 2011). Moreover mindfulness practice improves empathy and compassion (Mamgain, 2010). I also found some literature on contemplative practices for educators in terms of reducing their stress (Anderson, Levinson, Barker & Kiewra, 1999; Franco, Mañas, Cangas, Moreno & Gallego, 2010). My primary interest at that point was the effect of educators' mindfulness on their own education practice, which has had limited attention in the literature.

Following my decision to explore and incorporate mindfulness practice in teaching, I learnt that in teaching, as in MindBody healthcare, the teachers' ability to build relationship, their "capacity for connectedness" (Palmer, 2007, p. 11), and their "identity ... and integrity" (p. 14), are fundamental to transformation in the students' learning.

I discovered that in my anxiety about tertiary teaching in general I was trying to teach the students everything I thought they should know, i.e., the traditional "what subjects shall we teach" question (Palmer, 2007, p. 4). Additionally, because of my limited experience in tertiary teaching and my fear of the student group, I was, in a deep and semi-conscious way (Palmer, 1993) living out and exemplifying one of Palmer's maxims: "we teach who we are" (2007, p. 2). This was not what I had envisaged when applying for my position. I had struggled to think of how to build relationship within teaching environments, following my colleague's presentation (mentioned in the previous section) so I started to hold my teaching practice in awareness during my formal meditation sessions, and to practise informal mindfulness during preparation of teaching material and during class sessions.

Putting mindful education into practice

Since bringing mindfulness into my education practice, a number of things have changed. First, I am making a greater commitment to my own formal meditation practice. I support and encourage occupational therapy students to develop their practitioner intimacy skills (Broom, 1997) such as self-awareness, ability to be fully and authentically present in the therapeutic relationship, to sensitively challenge and at the same time be compassionate towards the person seeking healthcare assistance. This confirmed my growing understanding that I need to have that mindful presence, as well as intimacy skills, well developed in myself, in order to model this in the classroom. Darling Hammond stated that the first way of learning compassion in an educational context is through teacher modelling (Stanford University, 2010). Furthermore, Kabat-Zinn (2011) asserted that "mindfulness can only be understood from the inside out", i.e., through our own committed meditation practice, while recognising that "ultimately there is no inside and no outside, only one seamless whole" (p. 284), aligning it well with integrative MindBody practice.

What follows are some examples of the changes I experienced as a result of formal and informal mindfulness practice brought to bear on my teaching.

During a meditation while preparing for a teaching session I recognized I had been completely focused on the teaching material and was aware of a sense of "hiding behind the information" and trying to "disappear" myself. During another session I suddenly realised that I was simply trying to "get my head around the content" (personal journal entries, August 2011). On both occasions, the realisations created internal space and openness; I was able to be more present to the anxiety surrounding the preparations for the sessions, and go into the sessions more present to myself and to the students.

Second, in preparing the content and the structure of lesson material, I now limit the content to the most important information and allow space for reflection and exploration within the session on a regular basis, as supported by Brady (2007), and creating an opportunity for transformational learning (Duerr, Zajonc & Dana, 2003). This approach was in part inspired by a poem called *Fire* by Judy Brown (cited in Intrator & Scribner, 2003, p. 89), which refers to the need to include space between logs when building fires, as that is what enables a fire to burn. This is congruent with Dewey's argument that intellectual activity at its best becomes a "whole-hearted (experience that) … takes possession of us altogether" because "mental and bodily reactions are not two different things" (cited in Shusterman, 2008, p. 187). I am pleased with this development, as I would have felt too anxious earlier on to trust myself to be able to facilitate the learning process in this more contemplative way.

Third, in preparing myself for each teaching or facilitation session I create sufficient time and space to have at least a few minutes of quiet reflection time before the session starts. I centre myself, i.e., just noticing my breathing, my thoughts, my feelings, my body. The purpose of bringing mindful attention to my whole being is to note specific aspects as valuable information about what is going on for me in a given situation and respond in a way that is appropriate. My experiences described below are an example of that. My initial internal responses may be more symptoms of my emotions and the dynamic between me and the students, than solely a reflection of students' behaviour and attitudes.

My way of being and responding to students during sessions has changed considerably. I now make a concerted effort to learn students' names, in an attempt to address as many as possible by name, even within a lecture. Nugent (2011) identified learning students' names as one way of creating a safe emotional environment. A particular teaching session became a turning point; as I became more aware of my body, my sense of the student group, and the environment, it was as though suddenly the light went on, and I realized that I could see many individuals whose names I knew and with whom I did have a connection, in amongst the previously experienced sea of blank faces that had caused fear and anxiety.

I realize, like Southern (2007), that there is limited scope to focus on individual relationships with students in a lecture context, but that it is possible to develop a "learning community ... (in which to) ... hold the tension that opens the possibility for transformative learning ... (and) ... create a safe space for vulnerability" (p. 330) and exploration.

An example of this occurred during a tutorial as the class fell utterly silent and no one responded to my questions. I was aware of my discomfort about this and an inclination to get impatient and frustrated, and to want the group to interact. Instead I was able to take a few moments and wondered out loud: "I notice you have all gone silent and am not sure how to interpret this. I wonder what is going on." One or two students indicated they felt overwhelmed, then almost all others agreed and the flow of interaction was re-established.

Thus, I have recently come to understand and know from my experiences that my lived body has the potential not only to provide me with information about the impact of past experience on my current health status and personhood, but I have an opportunity to access information from all the dimensions of my lived body in the moment of experiencing it (not just through my accumulated theoretical, research or practice knowledge). This can only occur through bringing my own open-hearted mindful awareness to all of the multiple dimensions of myself and the other person(s) and of the interpersonal space. As described in the examples above, the information gained from that awareness can be utilized to respond in a way that facilitates the development of a respectful, compassionate, caring and enabling relationship, and an environment that allows for new learning to occur by all involved in the interaction, whether this is in a healthcare, an educational, or a collegial work context.

Conclusion

Developing a MindBody approach in my current work context has been complex, challenging and deeply satisfying at the same time. Consciously bringing an integrative MindBody awareness, spiritual qualities of being, lived body sensitivity and mindfulness into my role in occupational therapy education has started increasing my presence in lectures, my compassion for students, my ability to create a transformative learning community in the lectures and tutorials; and has led to a recovery of my confidence that I have something to offer because of who I am. There is still a lot to learn and develop, but I have made a solid start in fulfilling my yearning for a greater degree of integration between who I am as a person and who I am as an occupational therapist and educator. I can now wholeheartedly and from my own experience agree with Palmer that "every way of knowing becomes a way of living ... every epistemology becomes an ethic"(1993).

References

Anderson, V. L., Levinson, E. M., Barker, W. & Kiewra, K. R. (1999). The effects of meditation on teacher perceived occupational stress, state and trait anxiety, and burnout. *School Psychology Quarterly 14*: 3–25.

Astin, J. A., Shapiro, S. L., Lee, R. A. & Shapiro, D. H. (1999). The construct of control in mind-body medicine: Implications for healthcare. *Alternative Therapies in Health and Medicine, 5*: 42–47.

Booth, R. (2001). Mind-body common sense. *Advances in Mind-Body Medicine, 17*: 3–4.

Brady, R. (2007). Learning to stop, stopping to learn. *Journal of Transformative Education, 5*: 372–394.

Bridle, M. J. (1999). Are doing and being dimensions of holism? *The American Journal of Occupational Therapy, 53*: 636–639.

Broom, B. (1997). *Somatic illness and the patient's other story*. London: Free Association Books.

Broom, B. (2007). *Meaning-full disease: How personal experience and meanings cause and maintain physical illness*. London: Karnac.

Brown, K. W., Ryan, R. M. & Creswell, J. D. (2007). Mindfulness: Theoretical foundations and evidence for its salutary effects. *Psychological Inquiry, 18*: 211–237.

Christopher, J. C., Chrisman, J. A., Trotter-Mathison, M. J., Schure, M. B., Dahlen, P. & Christopher, S. B. (2011). Perceptions of the long-term influence of mindfulness training on counselors and psychotherapists: A qualitative inquiry. *Journal of Humanistic Psychology, 51*: 318–349.

Cole, M. B. & McLean, V. (2003). Therapeutic relationships re-defined. *Occupational Therapy in Mental Health, 19*: 33–56.

Cunningham, A. J. & Watson, K. (2004). How psychological therapy may prolong survival in cancer patients: New evidence and a simple theory. *Integrative Cancer Therapies, 3*: 214–229.

Didonna, F. (Ed.). (2009). *Clinical handbook of mindfulness*. New York: Springer.

Duerr, M., Zajonc, A. & Dana, D. (2003). Survey of transformative and spiritual dimensions of higher education. *Journal of Transformative Education, 1*: 177–211.

Finlay, L. (2001). Holism in occupational therapy: Elusive fiction and ambivalent struggle. *American Journal of Occupational Therapy, 55*: 268–276.

Franco, C., Mañas, I., Cangas, A. J., Moreno, E. & Gallego, J. (2010). Reducing teachers' psychological distress through a mindfulness training program. *The Spanish Journal of Psychology, 13*: 655–666.

Gethin, R. (2011). On some definitions of mindfulness. *Contemporary Buddhism, 12*: 263–279.

Gockel, A. (2010). The promise of mindfulness for clinical practice education. *Smith College Studies in Social Work, 80*: 248–268.

Goldstein, J. & Kornfield, J. (1987). *Seeking the heart of wisdom: the path of insight meditation*. Boston, MA: Shambhala.

Grabovac, A. D., Lau, M. A. & Willett, B. R. (2011). Mechanisms of mindfulness: A Buddhist psychological model. *Mindfulness*: 154–166.

Grossman, P., Kappos, L., Gensicke, H., D'Souza, M., Mohr, D. C., Penner, I. K. & Steiner, C. (2010). MS quality of life, depression, and fatigue improve after mindfulness training: a randomized trial. *Neurology, 75*: 1141–1149.

Gruman, J., Rovner, M. H., French, M. E., Jeffress, D., Sofaer, S., Shaller, D. & Prager, D. J. (2010). From patient education to patient engagement: Implications for the field of patient education. *Patient Education and Counseling, 78*: 350–356.

Hart, T. (2004). Opening the contemplative mind in the classroom. *Journal of Transformative Education, 2*: 28–46.

Hawtin, H. & Sullivan, C. (2011). Experiences of mindfulness training in living with rheumatic disease: An interpretative phenomenological analysis. *British Journal of Occupational Therapy, 74*: 137–142.

Hede, A. (2010). The dynamics of mindfulness in managing emotions and stress. *Journal of Management Development, 29*: 94–110.

Hemphill-Pearson, B. J. & Hunter, M. (1997). Holism in mental health practice. *Occupational Therapy in Mental Health, 13*: 35–49.

Hick, S. F. & Bien, T. (Eds.). (2008). *Mindfulness and the therapeutic relationship*. New York: Guilford Press.

Intrator, S. M. & Scribner, M. (Eds.). (2003). *Teaching with fire: Poetry that sustains the courage to teach*. Bainbridge Island, WA: Jossey-Bass.

Irving, J. A., Dobkin, P. L. & Park, J. (2009). Cultivating mindfulness in health care professionals: A review of empirical studies of mindfulness-based stress reduction (MBSR). *Complementary Therapies in Clinical Practice, 15*: 61–66.

Johnson, J. A. (1996). Occupational science and occupational therapy: An emphasis on meaning. In: R. Zemke & F. A. Clark (Eds.), *Occupational Science: The Evolving Discipline* (pp. 393–397). Philadelphia, PA: F.A. Davis.

Kabat-Zinn, J. (1996). *Full catastrophe living: How to cope with stress, pain and illness using mindfulness meditation* (new ed.). New York: Bantam Doubleday.

Kabat-Zinn, J. (2005). *Wherever you go there you are: Mindfulness meditation in everyday life* (10th anniversary ed.). New York: Hyperion.

Kabat-Zinn, J. (2011). Some reflections on the origins of MBSR, skillful means, and the trouble with maps. *Contemporary Buddhism, 12*: 281–306.

Kang, C. & Whittingham, K. (2010). Mindfulness: A dialogue between Buddhism and clinical psychology. *Mindfulness*: 161–173.

Kielhofner, G. (2009). *Conceptual foundations of occupational therapy practice* (4th ed.). Philadelphia, PA: F.A. Davis.

Kielhofner, G., Tham, K., Baz, T. & Hutson, J. (2002). Performance capacity and the lived body. In G. Kielhofner (Ed.), *Model of human occupation: Theory and application* (3rd ed., pp. 81–98). Philadelphia, PA: Lippincott Williams & Wilkins.

Lipton, B. (2005). *The biology of belief: Unleashing the power of consciousness, matter, and miracles.* Santa Rosa, CA: Mountain of Love/Elite Books.

Mamgain, V. (2010). Ethical consciousness in the classroom: How Buddhist practices can help develop empathy and compassion. *Journal of Transformative Education, 8*: 22–41.

Miller, J. P. (2006). *Educating for wisdom and compassion: Creating conditions for timeless learning.* Thousand Oaks, CA: Corwin Press.

Myss, C. & Shealy, N. (1999). *The creation of health: The emotional, psychological, and spiritual responses that promote health and healing.* London: Transworld Publishers.

Nagatomo, S. (1992). *Attunement through the body.* Albany, NY: State University of New York Press.

Nhat Hanh, T. (1987). *The miracle of mindfulness: An introduction to the practice of meditation* (M. Ho, Trans.). Boston, MA: Beacon Press.

Nugent, D. (2011). Teaching for learning. In N. Zepke, D. Nugent & L. Leach (Eds.), *Reflection to transformation: a self-help book for teachers* (2nd ed., pp. 81–98). Wellington, New Zealand: Dunmore Publishing.

Palmer, P. (1993). *The violence of our knowledge: Toward a spirituality of higher education.* Last accessed October 8, 2011, from http://wwkarios2.com/palmer_1999.htm

Palmer, P. (2007). *The courage to teach: exploring the inner landscape of a teacher's life* (10th anniversary ed.). San Francisco: Jossey-Bass.

Palmer, P., Zajonc, A., Scribner, M. & Nepo, M. (2010). *The heart of higher education: A call to renewal*. Last accessed October 8, 2011 from http://AUT.eblib.com.au/patron/FullRecord.aspx?p=547063

Parker, D. (2006). The client-centred frame of reference. In: E. A. S. Duncan (Ed.), *Foundations for practice in occupational therapy* (pp. 193–215). Edinburgh: Elsevier Churchill Livingstone, 2006.

Peloquin, S. M. (2002). Reclaiming the vision of reaching for heart as well as hands. *American Journal of Occupational Therapy, 56*: 517–526.

Pert, C. B., Dreher, H. E. & Ruff, M. R. (1998). The psychosomatic network: Foundations of mind-body medicine. *Alternative Therapies in Health and Medicine, 4(4)*: 30–41.

Reed, K., Hocking, C. & Smythe, E. (2010). The interconnected meanings of occupation: The call, being-with, possibilities. *Journal of Occupational Science, 17*: 140–149.

Roter, D. L., Stashefsky-Margalit, R. & Rudd, R. (2001). Current perspectives on patient education in the US. *Patient Education and Counseling, 44*: 79–86.

Shapiro, S. L., Brown, K. W. & Astin, J. (2011). Toward the integration of meditation into higher education: A review of research evidence. *Teachers College Record, 113*: 493–528.

Shusterman, R. (2008). *Body consciousness: A philosophy of mindfuness and somaesthetics*. New York: Cambridge University Press.

Siegel, D. (2007). *The mindful brain: Reflection and attunement in the cultivation of well-being*. New York: W.W. Norton.

Siegel, D. (2010). *The mindful therapist: A clinician's guide to mindsight and neural integration*. New York: W.W. Norton.

Silvester Clark, B. (n.d.). *Free your life*. Last accessed January 19, 2012, from http://www.freeyourlife.co.nz/FreeYourLife/About_Us.html

Southern, N. L. (2007). Mentoring for transformative learning. *Journal of Transformative Education, 5*: 329–338.

Stanfield, S. (2003). *The effects a transformational educational program, composed from the science of the mindbody continuum, has on the overall health and well-being of participants*. Unpublished doctoral dissertation. Holos University Graduate Seminary.Bolivar, MO. Last accessed January 19, 2012, fromhttp://holosuniversity.net/pdf/stanfieldDissertation.pdf

Stanford University. (2010, October 16). *The role of compassion in education and the wider societal context* (Video file). Last accessed January 19, 2012, from http://www.youtube.com/watch?v=S_xqCg2nIQ8

Stew, G. (2011). Mindfulness training for occupational therapy students. *British Journal of Occupational Therapy, 74*: 269–276.

Svenaeus, F. (2000). *The hermeneutics of medicine and the phenomenology of health: Steps towards a philosophy of medical practice.* Dordrecht, The Netherlands: Kluwer Academic.

Thera, N. (1996). *The heart of buddhist meditation.* San Francisco: Weiser Books.

Thompson, B. (2009). Mindfulness-based stress reduction for people with chronic conditions. *The British Journal of Occupational Therapy, 72:* 405–410.

Toombs, S. K. (1988). Illness and the paradigm of lived body. *Theoretical Medicine and Bioethics, 9:* 201–226.

Townsend, E. & Polatajko, H. (2007). *Enabling occupation II: Advancing an occupational therapy vision for health, well-being & justice through occupation.* Ottawa, Ontario: CAOT Publications ACE.

Wisneski, L. A. & Anderson, L. (2005). *The scientific basis of integrative medicine.* Boca Raton, FL: CRC Press.

Wood, W. (2004). The heart, mind, and soul of professionalism in occupational therapy. *American Journal of Occupational Therapy, 58:* 249–257.

Zajonc, A. (2009). *Meditation as contemplative enquiry: When knowing becomes love.* Great Barrington, MA: Lindisfarne Books.

CHAPTER FIFTEEN

Healing through talk and touch

Chris Cornelius

This is the story of my journey as a patient, a twenty year quest to experience healing from persistent, often debilitating, symptoms of an increasingly common chronic condition. Writing is a large part of my chosen profession, but this is one of the more difficult pieces of writing I have undertaken. I am a mid-career academic social scientist, specializing in matters of health systems and health policy. My story is given shape and colour by this professional background as I am inherently interested in how people get access to, and experience, health services. I still believe that these things are vitally important, but my story also demonstrates the limitations of seeking healing through medical care, and its various interventions and pharmaceutical treatments. I have a very positive experience of integrated MindBody work, and at the end of this Chapter I make a modest attempt to convey what the experience was like for me. However, another reason I want to tell this story is to relate, from a patient perspective, just how difficult it can be to find MindBody work, even though I had been primed for it for nearly twenty years.

I begin this story by providing some case notes; outlining my experience of diagnosis and treatment in the health care system from birth to my mid-forties. I do this in order to lay the foundations of my story; and to show the inherent difficulties and frustrations involved in making sense of my symptoms and experience within the confines of medical understanding. Though the details are unique, the overall pattern and shape of this experience, I believe, is increasingly common. In the middle section of the Chapter, I overlay my biographical details onto this biomedical narrative, setting the stage for the final part of the Chapter in which I convey my experience of the MindBody therapeutic process, which took the details of this biography seriously, and out of which healing became possible .

Navigating the health system with a chronic condition

Not long after my forty-third birthday, I was diagnosed with multiple food allergies and intolerances by an allergy specialist in a private clinic, and, at the time, it felt like an enormous mystery had been solved. My adult life had been dogged by bouts of severe eczema, and in my thirties I was hospitalized four times as skin infections ran out of control. I knew that there was a link between allergy and the three conditions of asthma, eczema and rhinitis; and I had suffered them all in various forms and combinations. I had multiple food allergies in childhood, and as an adult I knew to avoid foods that tended to exacerbate my symptoms. This diagnosis, in my forties, of "multiple food allergies and intolerances", felt like a revelation. The allergist said confidently that by eliminating problematic foods, and undergoing a programme of desensitization to environmental allergies, I should see a seventy to ninety percent improvement in my health. Initially, this prediction came true. I made great efforts to restrict my diet and my symptoms receded. However, by the next spring, six months into the new regime, they began to return, and the more I attempted to keep them under control, the more difficult the task seemed to become. After another year, my symptoms seemed worse than ever, with the added complication of feeling miserable about my food restrictions. It was very difficult to go out to a café or restaurant, or to invite guests for dinner. I felt like the walls were closing in on me.

My experience of this chronic condition of eczema goes back well before conscious memory. At about nine months of age, I was hospitalized with severe eczema. Family legend has it that I had my arms strapped down to prevent me from scratching. My earliest memories, however, are not of broken and weeping skin, but of shortness of breath and wheeziness with almost any physical exertion. Asthma was a constant school companion. When I was six years old, my father spent many sleepless nights in the lounge room, while I slept on a couch with the end above my feet propped up so that breathing would not be as difficult. The smell and taste of Intal, an asthma medication of the 1970s, breathed in as a bitter tasting powder through a rotating inhaler, will remain with me forever.

I also had a number of food allergies; something that seemed unusual, though not unheard of, at the time. Top of the list was peanut allergy, with egg and legumes as the other foods I knew I needed to avoid. The nausea and inevitable vomiting that went with any accidental ingestion of peanut were well and truly enough to keep me away from these foods. At primary school, eczema was not a large part of the picture, but this changed around the time I turned thirteen. As my teenage years progressed my eczema grew steadily worse; the rawness of skin behind my knees was constant. From what I can remember, visits to doctors mainly resulted in prescriptions for steroid creams.

Not long after my nineteenth birthday my eczema had become sufficiently severe for me to be referred to a hospital clinic, and so began my somewhat fraught relationship with the steroid wonder drug Prednisone. As a graduate student I studied in a city away from home and away from the family doctor, and for health care I moved between university health services and suburban general practitioners (GP). The main interaction with GPs and their nurses involved managing various eczema-related crises such as staphylococcal infections. Treatment commonly involved getting on to Prednisone with the intention of getting off as soon as was practicable. Over the years this became harder and harder to do. I cannot recall, through this time, whether any primary care practitioner ever talked about referral to medical specialists, but I was hardly in a position to afford the fees. I first visited a specialist dermatologist in my late twenties, and was told of new "miracle drugs" on the treatment horizon. The treatment remained one of steroid creams, moisturiser creams, and oral steroids and antibiotics to deal with the regular crises.

After completing my PhD, I took up my first academic position. I was now thirty, and had for the first time a reasonable income, so specialist dermatologist fees were no longer quite as daunting. By that time I was hardly ever off the oral steroid Prednisone; the best I could ever manage was to have 10 mg on alternate days. Accordingly, the specialist I consulted strongly advised me to wean myself off them due to the serious long-term side-effects. I did this, but without much of a backup plan. Consequently, I spiralled into seemingly never-ending bouts of staphylococcal infections, and few parts of my skin were free from active eczema. Those parts that were free were permanently red and dry, requiring multiple doses of moisturising cream every day.

Eventually, I was hospitalized for about two weeks. The hospital was a small suburban one close to the university where I worked. It was being used as an overflow hospital while the one up the road was undergoing renovation. At that time, the specialist skin ward had been temporarily relocated to the small campus. The legacy from that hospitalization was a frightening battle with the methicillin antibiotic-resistant staphylococcus bacterium, MRSA. Months of treatment with expensive alternative antibiotics ensued. Before the year was out, however, I was back in the skin ward for a further three weeks.

In the meantime I had agreed to take up a new job the following year, which required me to move cities again. Once there, I found a GP who handled my condition in similar ways to my previous experience; steroid creams, occasional Prednisone, and referral to a specialist dermatologist. This particular specialist was keen to offer hope in the form of powerful immunosuppressant medications. On his advice, I spent two to three years on Cyclosporin, most likely at great expense to the taxpayer. In any case, the treatment regime was not enough to prevent major outbreaks. After three years I was again hospitalized when the combination of a viral and bacterial staphylococcal infection became too much for my immune system. Another hospitalization followed a year later.

Two years after this, my fourth hospitalization, I made my first ever visit to an allergy specialist on the advice of a naturopath. This had never been suggested by my GP. I did not know such a specialty existed. My experience with secondary care has been one of good crisis management. None of the specialist clinicians I encountered before I consulted an allergy specialist had the time, inclination, or frame of mind, to start looking into what lies behind this chronic condition. Whatever clues I did pick up along the way were not picked up through my experience of allopathic health practitioners, and by my mid-twenties I had learnt not to expect anything different.

From the allergy specialist I received some information on my allergies, but no follow-up appointment. In any case, I had a couple of years in which my skin symptoms were less troublesome. However, before too long they became worse again. At around that time, an article appeared in a high circulation weekly magazine on food allergies that featured a specialist allergist. I had changed GPs by this time and one of the practitioners referred me to this specialist. Initially, this food allergy and intolerance diagnosis was a revelation, but after eighteen months, I visited my allergy specialist in desperation. In fact, this happened after I had asked the dietician in the practice to recommend a psychologist who could give some advice on how to cope with the enormously restricted diet. It was then that my specialist suggested I visit a colleague of his who was both an allergy specialist and psychotherapist; this was how I found my way to MindBody work. I went in a somewhat resigned spirit.

Overlaying biography onto biology?

I am the fourth and youngest child of parents who in the 1950s migrated from Europe to Australia. Three children were born within three years of arriving in their new country. During her third pregnancy, my mother was hospitalized for many months with tuberculosis. Over the next few years, she was beset by many anxieties, and a compulsion to keep the home free of germs and caring for three young children was very stressful. I strongly suspect that her pregnancy with me on top of all this was highly challenging for her. After I was born, she experienced quite severe post-natal depression.

My mother's anxieties and struggles profoundly shaped my early years. I have enduring memories of being a rather withdrawn child; fearful of physical activity, having few playmates, and stubbornly refusing to smile in family photos. I spent much of my time listening to the radio and playing solitary games. This, undoubtedly, is a selective and exaggerated picture. My father and siblings certainly gave me plenty of care, and my mother loved me very much, but I know she was suffering enormously.

When I was five, my mother took a holiday to visit her family in Europe. Once there, she could not bring herself to return. Eventually, after nearly a year away, she did so. However, on her return she became more withdrawn and agoraphobic, spending brief periods in a psychiatric hospital. After another year or so, when I was seven, she returned to Europe permanently. I remember vividly the day that we took her to the airport. I also remember (or perhaps was reminded of this much later by my mother) that I did not cry.

Just after I turned ten, my father remarried. Blended families were a rarity in my Catholic milieu, and there were few roadmaps available for the ride. It was not an easy experience for any of us, especially in the early years.

I moved out of home as soon as I completed high school. At eighteen I moved cities to work for a student organization inspired by ideals of social justice. From the day I arrived, however, I entered a fairly unrelenting spiral of self-doubt. I had few skills, and I doubted my capacity to live up to the ideals of the organization. I was in a big city, knew few people and became very depressed, but had little insight into this experience. After a little over a year, my life was increasingly dysfunctional and this was the period during which I checked into the hospital clinic with my first bout of very severe eczema since infancy. Soon after, I resigned my job and returned to my home city to the relative safety of a public service job. I started a Bachelor of Arts at university, which I thoroughly enjoyed, and then left work to study full-time. I had found what I loved and was soon pursuing graduate study. On the advice of some fellow students and teachers, I moved once again to a new city. This worked out well for me in the long term, and I stayed to do a PhD. However, the move also meant facing some of the demons arising from my earlier experience in a new city. The first two years were extremely tough; self-doubt returned and my health deteriorated.

At twenty-five, I had already been enrolled one year in a PhD. However, I knew it was time to visit my mother and meet my extended family in Europe. This was an extremely powerful experience. I was reunited with my mother after eighteen years. I spent five months in Europe, and for some of that time I stayed with one of my aunts. She was a social worker for a university hospital specializing in counselling people with skin conditions. She also knew much of my childhood story; she had visited our family when I was twelve. She also had known my mother and her family since childhood, and had been on hand for debriefing after my first visit to my mother. She was the first person to help forge a connection between my biography and my medical history.

I returned to my studies knowing that there was some work to do. Up until that point I had been frustrated with myself for not making the most of opportunities and abilities. I returned from Europe in a different headspace; knowing that in many ways it was remarkable I had survived as well as I had. I had been protected from having to deal with the realities and legacies of my early years until then, and I knew at that point that understanding and healing the legacies of my childhood was something I needed to do to relieve my ongoing suffering. There was no clear path to follow. As a student, I had limited resources, so the first significant step I took was to join a weekly dream discussion group. This was my first experience at attempting to recognize the powerful symbols and stories that lived beneath my conscious everyday reality. It helped me discover parts of myself; including one particular dream character that symbolized a very fearful and controlling part of me.

The next move for my first academic job marked a new phase of the story. In my first year I quickly developed a network of friends and felt optimistic and energized about the new part of my life. However, in my second year, everything seemingly solid turned to sand. Most of my social network moved away. I was asked to take over as lecturer of two courses after another staff member resigned. I felt desperately unprepared for this as the courses were in areas quite different from my PhD study. The early part of that year was quite turbulent for my family as well. At around that time, a gunman went on the rampage in a place that was very special for me; where our family had gone for holidays since I was six. Various family members and friends luckily managed to avoid being in the wrong place at the wrong time.

This perfect storm of stress and upheaval served to undermine my capacity to survive and function with my chronic eczema, and by August that year I was hospitalized. It was a surreal time and I have very few clear memories of it, other than trying to survive from day to day. This was also the year, co-incidentally, that I discovered massage therapy. I shared a house with a woman who was a very able massage therapist, and came to know the powerful effect it could have on me.

The following year I moved cities again to take up a new job. I was still rather fragile. Once again I was faced with making my way in a city in which I had no connections. My early years there were a struggle, but after three years I had become increasingly settled and able to look forward with some confidence. Two further hospitalizations showed me that I was still very vulnerable to external shocks, but there appeared to be light at the end of the tunnel.

I spent a period of academic research leave in the northern hemisphere. Once again I spent time with my mother, and with my aunt, reinforcing some of the connections made ten years earlier. Over the next two years, I launched into psychotherapy. I felt ready for a sustained process of work and with the help of my psychotherapist I made some important progress. I was able to tell my story, discover new insights and connections. Gradually, my health seemed to be improving. During that period, I met my future wife. The early years of our relationship were a wonderfully healing time. We married within a couple of years, and after another two years our daughter was born. One legacy of becoming a father, however, was that I downplayed the importance of my own physical wellbeing; finding it very hard to make the time to exercise. We renovated our house when our daughter was a toddler and, in retrospect, that was not great for my health, though the motive for doing it was the old carpet, which was heaven on earth for house dust mites. Not long after, my eczema and rhinitis had become seriously debilitating again. This was when I began to visit the private allergy specialist clinic, and finally was referred to a MindBody physician who was also an immunologist and a psychotherapist.

The MindBody experience

I came into MindBody work on a diet which was so restricted and such a drain on my energies that I often despaired. Interestingly, the food allergies I had long known about, nuts, eggs and shellfish, were not the major problem. The biggest restriction and the hardest thing to manage was my intake of salicylates, or natural aspirins, found widely in fruit and vegetables. Dining out felt almost impossible and I was very miserable. Despite the diet most of my skin was red, swollen, and very dry, as were my eyes. I needed to cover myself with aqueous cream two or three times a day. Whilst my eczema and rhinitis were challenging and worsening at this time, another symptom that seemed to be closely related to salicylate ingestion was even more distressing. Whenever I had gone over the recommended limit, or was close to it, I would burp uncontrollably. These were deep belches that seemed to come from deep within, and could be extremely uncomfortable and embarrassing.

From the beginning, my MindBody clinician challenged my recently acquired understanding that I was ultra-sensitive to food, or more particularly, that my symptoms were dependent on what I ate. Whatever the merits of the salicylate sensitivity diagnosis, it had given me a knowledge and belief that I should be now able to control my symptoms. Clearly that was not working very well. The work with the MindBody clinician was not so much about me finding out new things. I knew my story, had told it before, and had learned how to probe and question; but the process felt incomplete. I had some sense of a missing ingredient. At times, I would be describing some things that were harrowing but in a matter-of-fact way. I did feel things as I told my story, but the feelings were fleeting and elusive. I had very little language for them. My feelings came through my body, through itching, restlessness and belching. My words were measured, calibrated and controlled.

About three months into our work, we both came to a sense that talking, while helpful and necessary in communicating details of my story, was not enough in itself to lead to healing. My therapist had an intuition at this point, that some work involving touch just might be worth trying in conjunction with talk. He felt that my early story as an infant suggested that there had not been enough soothing touch and that continuing talk therapy on its own was ironically maintaining the ancient status quo. He referred me to a massage therapist and I was very happy to take up this suggestion. After all, in the late 1990s regular massage therapy was the one thing that seemed to calm me down and offer some very temporary relief and respite. However, it was one of many things that was low on my list of priorities once I became a father; it was a luxury (of time mainly) that I could not afford.

About ten minutes into my second massage session, I began to burp uncontrollably; this then transformed into an enormous emotional release. I cried for the remainder of the session; but I knew that what was happening was a release of feeling that had been frozen in my body for a long, long time. These feelings remain difficult to put into words. At their core is a deep sadness about my mother mixed with a child's sense that I was the cause of her having to leave. Most likely, they go back to a prevailing sense I believe I had from infancy that my mother suffered because I existed. I look back on that day and see it as the turning point, the pivotal moment in a process that involved many sessions with my MindBody and massage therapists.

Of course, talking, and talking through the touch experiences were still important. What I knew now was that much of what had previously been inexpressible, other than through my skin, had now found another way to be released. With the two modes, talk and touch, working in tandem, I began to feel that I had found a path out of my prison. Apart from that one massage therapy session, there were no further moments of catharsis. There was, however, in one MindBody talk session, one very striking revelation, which took me completely by surprise.

In the winter of 2010, during the course of my therapy, I and my family spent a couple of days in a sleepy village a couple of hours from home. In a second hand bookshop I spotted a copy of *Cat's Eye* by Margaret Atwood (1993). I had read and loved others of her books and so had no hesitation in snapping up this one. It is a book about a woman, Elaine, in her fifties; a successful artist returning to Toronto, the city in which she grew up. She has avoided returning to Toronto for some time, and experiences a feeling of dread; particularly of meeting a childhood friend. This story is interwoven with her partial recollections of childhood in which Elaine was nearly killed as the result of a rather malicious childhood prank that had gone wrong, instigated by the friend whom she later dreads meeting. Elaine nearly dies of hypothermia, having been trapped in an icy river; but as a child she is unable to make sense of this and the damage done finds other ways of manifesting in later life.

I started relating this in one talk session, because this part of the book had touched a deep nerve. Apart from the superficial parallels between my story and Elaine's (of childhood trauma that was too much to deal with) what this story gave me was a metaphor that deeply resonated. This was the metaphor of ice. There were things that I could not express as a child; instead my well of feeling became frozen. I had always known this ice was there, but it could not flow through me and out of me. I understood then that it was possible to poke and prod at frozen emotions, to know one's way around them; that is what I could do when I talked. However, the ice needed to thaw in order for me to experience the power of those emotions in my body. This story provided me with a metaphor for what had happened in my second massage session; an experience of breaking through the ice.

I look back on this experience of MindBody work and see it as quite an amazing journey. I had struggled for twenty years. Much of that time I experienced little progress and there were many dead ends. Many times I even forgot that it was important. I had always assumed that it was not possible to find a way of working that brought together biography and biology. While my aunt's career in Europe indicated that such work happened somewhere in the world, I never found anything equivalent in Australasia. Few conventional medical practitioners, in my experience, were able to help me along the way. Of course, there were many practitioners I sought, more from the complementary/ alternative end of the clinical spectrum, who believed in the intricate relationship between the physical and the emotional; but they could never get to the level of specificity that would help to join the dots. It just might be that I needed twenty years in the wilderness to find the right combination. What I feel I have gained through this process has not come easily, which makes it all the more precious. Maybe it was necessary for me to undertake a lengthy journey. In accepting this, I don't really have much anger at the failures of the health system and medical practice.

I have now experienced well over two years of very good health. While my symptoms have not gone entirely, they are now very manageable. Their volume and intensity have decreased considerably. I have never felt healthier for such a prolonged period of time. I have not been cured but I can claim to have experienced healing. The technologies of healing were voices and hands; nothing more than that.

Reference

Atwood, M. (1993). *Life before man/Cat's eye*. London: Bloomsbury.

CHAPTER SIXTEEN

Holding it all together: integrating the MindBody approach as a breast cancer patient

Peta Joyce

The story

As soon as our family doctor phoned and asked that my husband and I come and see him immediately, I knew. "I'm sorry", he said, "your biopsy shows breast cancer." He paused, and looking directly at me he said, "We all have to contemplate our mortality some time, and now here is your opportunity." I went immediately into what I now recognize as my "brave, coping self" and stepped up to his challenge, but I remember nothing of the rest of the interview; in truth I was in shock. I had no family history of cancer, and a supposedly clear mammogram one year before when I found a small lump in my right breast. Subsequently I could feel the lump was growing, and now the biopsy confirmed cancer.

The major and immediate emotional response to my diagnosis was fear; raw, chaotic, overwhelming fear. At the time this fear was hard to name, but later I recognized it as the fear of death, of the unknown, and of the medical system.

> Fear, how do I befriend you
> Unwelcome companion of the waiting hours

Of crisp white coats and polished corridors
Awakener of the reptile brain
Panic fluttering like drowning butterflies
Inside me
Coursing through my veins
Stalking me at unexpected turns
Uninvited companion of the dawn light chill
Show me your face
That I may stare into your eyes
And see my soul

(Joyce, 2008)

The grief was unexpected and powerful; about developing a serious illness, the possibility of dying and leaving loved ones. I had a strong identity as a healthy person. Having cancer challenged who I thought I was, and my ability to be in tune with my body, and my intuitive knowing. How could I have a serious health condition and not know on some level? My trust in my body and my self-knowledge was severely shaken.

I experienced deep shame about having cancer, especially as I am a health practitioner. I was challenged by a popular belief in the ability to be in charge of one's destiny and by a sense of failure if I did not manifest the desired reality. All this was a very short step from believing I created my own cancer, a perspective supported by a large body of self-help literature; and with an associated imperative to heal myself. Yet, although my beliefs and life choices may have contributed to my health situation, I feel these are over-simplified and individualistic views, which do not take into account the complex interplay between the personal, social, historical, physical and spiritual dimensions. Rebuilding my identity became a major task;

Map shatters on the anvil of fear
Pick up the pieces one by one
Broken shards of old belief
A new mosaic emerging

(Joyce, 2008)

I did not want to take on the identity of a cancer patient or a cancer survivor (in other words, to be defined by my illness) and I did not want others to relate to me differently because of their assumptions about me as a person with cancer. Using the resources of the Cancer Society or similar groups was difficult in this regard, because for me it reinforced the "person with cancer" identity. Other peoples' stories, although deeply humbling and sometimes inspirational, mainly triggered my fears. These organizations are very helpful for some people, but other than utilizing their counselling and massage services, they were not empowering for me. In fact, the breast cancer support industry largely reinforces a particular gender stereotype with its pink bows, sentimentality, and "Look Good Feel Better" programs; sugar coating and normalizing the experience of breast cancer without questioning its causes or treatment (Ehrenreich, 2002). I found the prevailing imperative to maintain a positive attitude throughout my cancer treatment difficult and relentless. It made me feel as though having the full gamut of my feelings was not legitimate; it seemed to be a denial of the reality of cancer, its treatment, and uncertain prognosis.

The three months waiting between diagnosis and surgery was agonizing. There was no knowing what stage the cancer was at or how contained it was. All I had was the biopsy. After meeting with the surgeon, I was left with a decision to have either a partial mastectomy and radiation, or a full mastectomy and no radiation. I was assigned a breast nurse, who was to be my first point of contact in case of any concerns. She was attentive and kind, and sent me away with calm reassurances and some very basic and general literature to read. If I tried to explore my options with her, her responses continued to be kind reassurances of the "surgeon knows best" type rather than an intelligent, informed discussion of the research and possible outcomes of the different options. There was no one in the public health system I could have this type of discussion with except my general practitioner (GP). It was an extremely challenging decision. I felt ill-equipped to make it. In the end, I used research via the internet, my GP and a counsellor to help me decide to have a partial mastectomy.

Surgery revealed two other health conditions, possible lymphoma and amyloidosis, that needed further investigation involving six specialists; surgeon, oncologist, haematologist, anaesthetist, radiologist and cardiologist. Were they each aware of my situation and conferring with one another? Did they understand the possible effects of breast cancer treatment on the other two conditions? Were the conditions all connected in some way? It seemed to me there was no-one in the medical system looking at how the different conditions might interact or be part of a bigger picture. I felt lost in a world I knew virtually nothing about, having had very little need of medical services over the years. Faced with making crucial decisions about treatment, when each specialist could only give me information about their own particular area, I was sailing alone in uncharted waters.

I desperately needed someone to hold the big picture for me, someone who had the medical expertise to encompass the range of health conditions I was facing and talk me through the treatment options. How was I to navigate my way through the medical maze and make decisions about what was right for me? How could I get the answers to my questions about the different medical diagnoses and how they were linked?

In addition to information about diagnosis and decisions about treatment, I needed to be engaged in my own healing, which was much more than simply accepting treatment and hoping it worked. I wanted to approach my healing from a unitary, or holistic, perspective. In my practice as a Holistic Pulsing bodymind therapist and teacher, I was very familiar with the concept of body as story; that our history and beliefs are embodied in our cells and expressed in our physical structure and ways of being (Browning, 1990, 2004). Through the unitary perspective "we are led to radical new understandings of disease, the simultaneity of mind and body, and the nature of reality" (Broom, 2002, p. 18). Healing involves a contextual fabric interwoven with the belief systems of the client and practitioner, the relationship between them, the wider support systems, and the historical, cultural, social and spiritual milieu in which healing takes place. In contrast to the unitary approach, the dualistic approach sees humans as being discrete and separate parts or aspects, which make up the whole. Healing is an external event where clients are seen as passive recipients of diagnosis and treatment administered to them by experts. This model still underpins many approaches to health, including conventional medicine and some fields of complementary medicine.

I needed to understand my cancer from a different perspective, one that acknowledged who I was historically, socially and culturally, and to access knowledge systems other than the conventional scientific paradigm. I needed someone who could embrace the emotional, mental and spiritual dimensions of my healing as well as the physical. I found no one person who could do this, although my GP, who is also an anthroposophical doctor, certainly encompassed a much wider view of illness and treatment than usual.

Roads to healing

Vaughan (2005) distinguishes three ways of knowing: sensory empiricism, rational analysis, and contemplative knowing. On the one hand, I wanted to surrender to the accumulated scientific knowledge and experience of medical specialists, accepting their rational analysis. On the other hand, I needed to be in touch with my own knowing, and make decisions that felt right for me. I began to use my gut reactions. The more I noticed my embodied response to different medical interviews, the more I noticed that they could be categorized as heartful or fearful; essentially reactions of love or fear. Eventually my decisions were partially guided by this gut reaction, a sensory empiricism; but it took courage to trust this knowing and not be overwhelmed by the biomedical paradigm, or driven by fear.

I found inner processes such as guided visualization, mindfulness meditation and reflection (Vaughan's contemplative knowing) useful for accessing my own deep internal wisdom. Attending to my subconscious mind was of paramount importance; for example, exploring more deeply my embodied and intuitive feelings about whether to have a full or partial mastectomy. Approaching this decision with my rational mind only left me with nightmares and uncertainty. I still do not know if having a partial mastectomy was the right decision, but it was the one I chose from the perspective of my inner and embodied wisdom, with the help of a counsellor who specializes in helping people facing major medical challenges (Silvester-Clark, Marsh & Stanfield, 2012). This type of inner work was deeply sustaining and comforting to me, and ultimately enabled me to come to a very different place in my approach to treatment.

To do this inner work, I used a range of practitioners and processes: counsellors, a hypnotherapist, a naturopath, bodywork, a poetry retreat, a family constellation workshop, a Process workshop involving ancestral healing, a series of body-casting sessions and Brandon Bay's Journey work (Bays, 1999). My long-term women's group gave me the space to express my raw emotions and helped me name, hold, and process what I was going through, as well as making meaning of my experience.

The dualistic perspective is often evident in choosing health interventions. Commonly, either conventional medicine or complementary approaches are favoured, often in opposition to each other. My own belief, prior to diagnosis, was that faced with a serious illness I would choose only natural or complementary medicine. The reality was very different. During inner work to access a wise aspect of myself, I came to a surprising realization, enabling me to accept and integrate both complementary and medical approaches. From my journal: "… all is useful; allopathic, complementary, natural, physical, emotional, energetic, spiritual, use it all. All approaches have the energy of light, of god, of divine life-force, everything under the sun is from source, just interpreted in different ways … whether people are from your belief system or not, all are motivated for good." A large part of my journey became confronting my fears of the medical system and my own dualistic thinking.

Inner work helped me to understand that reframing the fear as a symptom or call to action was a useful and empowering response, eventually allowing me to be with my feelings and accept them as a natural part of the process.

> This dance with fear
> Is a knife-edge
> Between surrender and self-knowing
> Fear and love,
> Who am I
> But a reed in the wind
> Swaying to my own music

(Joyce, 2008)

A Foreign Land

I had never been in hospital before, except to give birth or visit others, and it was a strange and alienating experience, like being in another world, with its own language, customs, hierarchies, and culture. My initial response was to become obedient and passive, to give myself over to perceived authority, just as I might in school or the legal system. My university studies in anthropology and sociology helped; I approached surgery as a process of initiation into a new culture and found ways to make it more empowering for me, such as visualizing healthy outcomes, making specific requests for appropriate statements to be read while under anaesthetic, and listening to calming music (through my Ipod).

> Three o'clock and all's well,
> The bright corridors have yielded their expertise,
> I am through the portal to the other side
> In the blink of an eye,
> Three hours have passed
> My body floats in smooth white cotton,
> Relieved and curious
> Unknown faces blur in and out of focus,
> Denizens of this world of metal-wheeled beds
> Machines measuring vital signs
> Citizens with strange language and customs,
> At last, a familiar face
> The surgeon, smiling, confident
> Her skills have delivered their magic
> A sacrifice to the cancer god

(Joyce, 2008)

Contextualizing surgery as a ritual process may seem far-fetched, but it helped me to make meaning of a foreign and potentially frightening and powerless experience by reframing it in a way I could relate to. Seeing the whole process as a rite of passage helped me to let go of old patterns and beliefs and to integrate a new way of being.

> I walk through a new portal
> Into the unknown
> Take this piece of beloved breast
> As a token of my dying to the past
> Take these cells that multiply too fast
> As a sacrifice to the busy, too-caring life
> Lay the knife upon my body
> With care for the woman within
> Who roars forth from the wound

To stamp her new life
Upon the bones of the old

(Joyce, 2008)

Surgery was actually easy to reframe as a rite of passage, with the hospital stay being a removal from everyday life, and the anaesthetic inducing an altered state of consciousness. Welch (2003) sees parallels between the practice of western medicine and ritual, and Achterburg (1992) points to the role of physicians as ritual makers at many of life's major passages. Young and Koopsen (2005) include prayer, meditation, visualization and guided imagery, gratitude, time in nature, art, and storytelling as examples of contemporary rituals used in other forms of healthcare. I certainly benefited from many of the above approaches, which I found spiritually satisfying and emotionally calming.

Client/practitioner relationship

Over and over again, whether with doctors or complementary therapists, how each clinician related to me had a huge impact on how I felt about treatment, my confidence in it, how I felt about myself as a person, and the choices I made.

The interview with the surgeon was a positive experience. She was efficient, but worked patiently through my long list of questions, being honest when she did not know the answer. I talked to her about my belief in the importance of the subconscious mind, and she responded willingly to my request for a positive statement about the surgery being read while I was under anaesthetic, and to my using my IPod during surgery, in a practical and matter of fact way. She was willing to accommodate my requests, which helped me feel accepted as an individual with particular needs, who was able to take some power in an otherwise powerless situation.

To my delight the anaesthetist doing the pre-operative assessment was completely in accord with my views on the bodymind and working with the subconscious. I have since discovered that his passion is bringing caring and compassion back into healthcare, and treating patients as whole beings (Youngson, 2012). Unfortunately he was not the anaesthetist on duty during my surgery, but he brought a further sense of connection and of being understood and accepted, into the otherwise alien environment of the hospital.

Surgery itself did not hold any great fear for me, but radiation was a very different matter. I went to the appointment with the radiotherapist with lots of questions, undecided about whether to proceed with treatment. He was very unforthcoming, came up with stock answers to my questions that did not take my individual circumstances into account, and could barely make eye contact with me. I left with a very bad feeling in the pit of my stomach, determined to do more research. The waiting list in Auckland was so long, I was eventually offered treatment in Hamilton or Sydney. The booking clerk was surprised I chose Hamilton; "women love the shopping in Sydney", she said cheerily. Leave my home and support networks and travel to another country for six weeks of radiotherapy, to enjoy the shopping? Clearly there are many different approaches to healing.

At the meeting with the Hamilton radiotherapist, I was by now quite defensive, and started the interview with: "You'll have to persuade me that this is the right thing to do". "I'm not here to persuade you", he said, "but to give you the information so that you can choose". We had a long and interesting discussion about the latest research on type and length of dose, and he agreed to vary the standard dose for a smaller amount over a shorter time frame, based on a large world-wide study he had just reviewed for his team and pulled then and there out of his pocket. I felt totally different; I had been listened to, treated like an intelligent human being who could make her own decisions, and left feeling positive about proceeding with radiation treatment.

The oncologist was a good listener, who did his best to give the information I asked for and look at my whole diagnosis, but mostly I felt the answers to my questions about medical treatment and prognosis were based on the clinician's own biases, or the current "stock" answer, rather than sensing the doctor was addressing my particular circumstances. The answers became predictable. For example, I knew from my research that the effects of exposure to radiation are cumulative. I had been exposed to many x-rays because of having double pneumonia as a child, and regular chest x-rays as a young adult, not knowing they could be harmful. I wanted to know what the possible long term effects of radiation treatment would be for me personally, but I never received other than a standard reassuring response about safe doses. It would have been so much more helpful and empowering to have had my questions at least acknowledged, and to be able to talk with someone willing to either do some research or support me to do it myself, or even to say with honesty, "we don't know the answer". For me, information is empowering, but on the whole, specific information about my medical condition was only given sporadically and practitioners were reluctant to be honest about the extent of their knowledge. For example, I needed follow-up surgery, because the margin between the tumour and healthy tissue from the initial surgery was too small for certainty; but it took several follow-up visits and questioning to find out that the second surgery showed tissue completely free of cancer cells. Being told "your results are all fine" is not enough for me. I need to know what that specifically means. I am still, four years on, getting new information from the haematologist in my follow-up visits—information she may well have given me at the outset, but which I do not remember.

Far from wasting time, honest, open and detailed communication would have built a better therapeutic relationship and could improve the outcome for me as a patient. Much research points to the positive correlation between a good therapeutic relationship and therapeutic outcome, and the importance of client choice (Lebow, 2006). Scovern (2003) concludes that factors in the patient, the physician, and in their interaction increase the effectiveness of conventional medical treatment by increasing compliance, improving the client's subjective state of wellbeing, and have direct psychophysiological effects. In a review of the research on the psychological aspects of MindBody medicine with cancer patients, researchers concluded that such interventions could improve quality of life, alter immune functioning and possibly survival rates (Simonton-Atchley & Sherman, 2005).

Symbols, meaning and the life journey

I was struck by how often the language used around cancer was symbolic of warfare. People with the disease were spoken of as heroes who fought or lost their battle with cancer. My healing involved preparing my body for surgery, and letting go of the tissue to be removed in a loving and respectful way; rather than merely cutting out the offending cells. Surgical removal of my tumour was a sensible (though paradoxical) part of a much wider approach. Creating and decorating a plaster cast of my torso during body-casting sessions (before I knew whether I would lose the whole or part of my breast) became a deeply symbolic, contemplative and self-loving process. The proliferating cells were a part of me, not to be removed but to be worked with to restore balance and wholeness. During a powerful visualization, I experienced the cancer cells as chaotic and random, trying to raise the energetic resonance or vibration of my body to live life more fully. A potent healing symbol became the koru (the stylized spiral shape of the unfolding tree-fern) where the cancer cells were lovingly contained and transformed within the curled fronds.

I became acutely aware of the power of visual symbols. During radiation therapy, being alone in a large vault-like room with its huge thick walls, strange machine, and "danger, radiation" symbols everywhere was a frightening experience. Imagine my delight to find a sunny beach scene painted on one wall, complete with real pebbles, deckchair and bucket and spade. Instead of imagining my body bombarded with dangerous radiation, I could visualize the healing rays of the sun as I lay on the beach. When I shared my appreciation for the mural with the staff, they told me the managers were going to have it removed to create a more corporate atmosphere.

Broom (1997, 2002, 2007), Welch (2003) and others point out the importance of the symbolic nature of illness and the meaning that patients make of their disease. The meaning of disease can be seen from a dualistic-warfare view of being under attack, or as an inevitable and natural part of the evolutionary process (Peters, 2006). Pelletier (2002) observes that in MindBody approaches, healing "does not exist 'outside' the individual, independent of 'inside' changes in attitude, lifestyle, and orientation toward self and environment." (p. 5). My approach to healing involved engaging my inner world, making sense and meaning of my disease, and contextualizing it as a part of my whole life journey.

Cancer for me was not a one-off event, but the culmination of a number of factors, including the recent death of both parents, three months of pneumonia, and moving house after twenty-two years. I discovered unconscious beliefs, some inherited, that were not conducive to my health, and psychological and emotional needs I was not attending to. It was important to discover the particular significance of breast cancer for me, to really listen to what my body was telling me. When I look back at my journals, I was already confronting the same life issues and patterns when I had pneumonia the year before; cancer was a continuation of the same process of realization and healing. True to a lifelong pattern of coping with every situation I was disregarding my own needs for nurturing and self-care in order to contend with major life events. The irony of now having to hold it all together in terms of an integrative approach to my healing was not lost on me.

For me, the journey was not just about a biomedical process of curing the breast cancer, but about healing the many dimensions involved in getting breast cancer in the first place, and in preventing its reoccurrence. Apart from my naturopath and GP, no-one in the medical system gave me any information about the possible precursors to, or subsequent prevention of, breast cancer, or any lifestyle changes I could make. The oncologist did prescribe a preventative drug, and was supportive of my decision not to take it (according to him it would have had "minimal benefit" in my case), but we did not discuss any other aspects of wellbeing. In contrast, I had a truly holistic healing experience during a week's residential retreat at The Monastery, near Hamilton. I was offered advice on nutrition, wellbeing and physical exercise, sessions of psychotherapy, meditation and mindfulness, massage and anthroposophical treatment, and given delicious nutrient-dense meals with ingredients from the organic garden. All this was offered in a sense of loving service, attention to detail and tailored to my individual needs.

The biomedical model sees healing as an external event, ignoring the effect of the client's inner world and the complex inter-subjective interplay between client, practitioner, and the environment. The MindBody approach sees all these aspects as important in healing. As Hirshberg (2005, p. 160) says, "The crisis of cancer and the realization of mortality awaken the desire to discover and understand who we really are, to take control of our lives, to believe we can influence the outcome." I was determined to be an active participant in, rather than a passive recipient of, medical intervention and to engage every aspect of myself as a whole person to facilitate healing. When I paid careful attention to what was around me, I was amazed at how often just the right person, book, workshop or resource turned up; how my whole environment supported healing.

This makes it sound easy. It was not. The journey was full of ups and downs and I really struggled to stay in the bodymind paradigm, true to what was right for me. It was very easy to give up and surrender to the dualistic paradigm and become a typical patient. The medical system on the whole was an alien, impersonal environment that deeply challenged my sense of uniqueness and personhood, my right to make informed choices and to see myself as a whole person rather than as a diagnosis or as having parts to be fixed. This is a critique of the system, not the individuals within it, who I sincerely believe are all working hard in their own, necessarily limited, ways in the best interests of their patients. Having to hold the bodymind perspective and the bigger health picture for myself was often overwhelming on top of everything else. It took a great deal of outside help and personal resourcefulness to come to any degree of physical, emotional or spiritual wellness.

There are interventions that the medical system could make which would facilitate whole person wellness to a much greater extent than it presently does. In my particular case, the time between diagnosis and treatment (both surgery and radiation) could have been greatly eased if I had been able to discuss treatment options with someone knowledgeable who also saw me as a whole person with my own unique life history, beliefs and ways of being. Getting honest answers and specific information where I asked for it would also have helped me to make more informed decisions and to feel empowered and partnered in my healing journey. With hindsight, I could have been more assertive and questioning where I did not get the help or information I needed; but that would have taken a great deal more energy and strength than I had at the time.

Conclusion

Ultimately, being with myself in all my chaotic and raw emotional turmoil, listening to myself deeply, living the journey fully and engaging spiritually with rebuilding my identity became a transcendent experience.

> In the face of fear and loss
> I taught myself gratitude
> Listening deeply to what is
> Rather than what was, or could be
> Savouring each moment
> For its luminous presence
> I came to know each bird in my garden
> The rhythms and habits of bees and insects
> Spent hours in contemplation of a single flower
> Lost myself in wonder at the changing patterns of sky, wind
>   and sea,
> Gazed at the night and felt the breath of dawn on my cheek

Opened my heart to the gift of loved ones, food and shelter
Life pared down to its everyday existence
And the simple, delicious, miracle of being alive

(Joyce, 2008)

Schlitz (2005, p. xl) defines integral medicine as "a dynamic, holistic, life-long process that exists in widening and deepening relationships with self, culture, and nature. Integral medicine is about transformation, growth, and the restoration of wholeness." The "restoration of wholeness" was, and still is, my primary focus. I have learned from experience that wholeness is not an achieved state, but an on-going process. The journey was unique to me, and not a recipe for healing.

Have I come to terms with my mortality, as my GP suggested? I have stared mortality in the face and, in the process, learned a great deal about myself and my loved ones. I am well, and being nearly five years down the track now, the prognosis is apparently good. I am learning about the power of living in the present, of not taking anything for granted, and the joy of gratitude. I am still fearful of a possible lingering painful decline before death, but not of dying itself. I still get triggered into fear, for example during follow-up visits about my ongoing, but completely stable, health conditions. The journey has been less about cure and more about meaning and living in each moment. The experience has been truly transformative, perhaps in spite of the medical system, rather than because of it.

References

Achterburg, J. (1992). Ritual: the foundation for transpersonal medicine. *ReVision, 14(3)*: 158–164.

Bays, B. (1999). *The Journey*. London: Thorsons.

Browning, T. (1990). *Gentle miracles*. Chatswood, Australia: Global Embrace.

Browning, T. (2004). *The power of softness: Holistic pulsing*. Kidron, Israel: Innana.

Broom, B. (1997). *Somatic illness and the patient's other story. A practical integrative mind/body approach to disease for doctors and psychotherapists.* London: Free Association Books.

Broom, B. (2002). Somatic metaphor: A clinical phenomenon pointing to a new model of disease, personhood, and physical reality. *Advances in Mind-Body Medicine, 18(1)*: 16–29.

Broom, B. (2007). *Meaning-full disease: How personal experience and meanings cause and maintain physical illness*. London: Karnac.

Ehrenreich, B. (2002). Welcome to Cancerland. In: S. J. Gould (ed.), *The best American essays*, (pp. 66–87). Boston: Houghton Mifflin Company, 2002.

Hirshberg, C. (2005). Living with Cancer: From Victim to Victor, the Integration of Mind, Body and Spirit. In: M. Schlitz, T. Amorok & M. Micozzi (Eds.), *Consciousness and healing: Integral approaches to mind-body medicine* (pp. 156–173). St Louis, MO: Elsevier Churchill Livingstone, 2005.

Joyce, P. (2008). Unpublished manuscript.

Lebow, J. (2006). *Research for the psychotherapist: from science to practice*. New York: Routledge.

Pelletier, K. (2002). Mind as healer, mind as slayer: MindBody medicine comes of age. *Advances 18(1)*: 4–15.

Peters, K. (2006). Spiritual transformation and healing in light of an evolutionary theology. In: J. D. Koss-Chioino & P. Hefner (Eds.), *Spiritual transformation and healing: Anthropological, theological, neuroscientific, and clinical perspectives* (pp. 134–151). New York: Altamira, 2006.

Schlitz, M. (2005). The integral impulse: The emerging model for health and healing. In: M. Schlitz, T. Amorok & M. Micozzi (Eds.), *Consciousness and healing: Integral approaches to mind-body medicine* (p. xl). St Louis, MO: Elsevier Churchill Livingstone, 2005.

Scovern, A. W. (2003). From placebo to alliance: The role of common factors in medicine. In: M. A. Hubble, B. L. Duncan & S. D. Miller (Eds.), *The heart and soul of change: What works in therapy.* (pp. 259–295). Washington, DC: American Psychological Association, 2003.

Simonton-Atchley, S. & Sherman, A. (2005). Psychological aspects of mind-body medicine: Promises and pitfalls from research with cancer patients. In: M. Schlitz, T. Amorok & M. Micozzi (Eds.), *Consciousness and healing: Integral approaches to mind-body medicine* (pp. 79–92). St Louis, MO: Elsevier Churchill Livingstone, 2005.

Sylvester-Clark, B., Marsh, R. & Stanfield, S. (2012). *Having surgery? Prepare well to recover well using the power of your mind*. Last accessed 20/08/2012. www.holistichealthmadesimple.com

Vaughan, F. (2005). Multiple ways of knowing. In: M. Schlitz, T. Amorok & M. Micozzi (Eds.), *Consciousness and healing: Integral approaches to mind-body medicine* (pp. 391–396). St Louis, MO: Elsevier Churchill Livingstone, 2005.

Welch, J. S. (2003). Ritual in western medicine and its role in placebo healing. *Journal of Religion and Health, 42(1)*: 21–33.

Young, C. & Koopsen, C. (2005). *Spirituality, health, and healing*. Sudbury, MA: Jones and Bartlett.

Youngson, R. (2012). *Time to care—how to love your patients and your job*. Raglan, New Zealand: Rebelheart.

CHAPTER SEVENTEEN

Transforming a pain clinic: using patient stories to integrate medical practice

Chris Hayes and Stephanie Oak

The telling of stories invites transformation from what we have been to what we are becoming. "If the clinical story is well told, it can enfold the pain story and save it from chaos. The pain may not go away. But pain can become something that is not antithetical to flourishing" (Frank, 2005). This account is built upon a foundation of many individual patient stories, yet it is also the story of reshaping a pain clinic and its influence within a broader healthcare system.

Hunter Integrated Pain Service (HIPS) is a multidisciplinary unit that services the acute and chronic pain needs of the people of the Hunter New England region of Australia, just north of Sydney. The referral area covers over 130,000 square kilometres (approximately the size of England) and has a population of 840,000. The unit is part of a large teaching hospital that is affiliated with the University of Newcastle. It is publicly funded and all services are free to patients after referral from their family doctor or other treating specialist.

HIPS was established in 1997 in response to the recognition that many of the pain presentations within the hospital system were chronic and complex, and did not respond to standard acute pain management strategies that were primarily biomedical in nature and designed around quick patient turnover. From the outset the Director of HIPS

(Chris Hayes), an anaesthetist, wanted to establish a service that could offer more than biomedical interventions, recognizing that the needs of patients with chronic pain were very different from those with acute pain. The clinical team included anaesthetists, rehabilitation physicians, nurses, physiotherapists, psychologists and a liaison psychiatrist (Stephanie Oak), and it aimed to provide a holistic model of care that was biopsychosocially focused for patients with acute cancer and persistent non-cancer pain.

It has taken these clinicians more than a decade to meet the challenges and resistances of a system that is firmly embedded in Western biomedicine. We have only just reached a point where the HIPS model of practice can truly be seen as holistic. This chapter describes the challenges we have faced in developing an integrated and multi-dimensional pain service, that aims to treat the person in pain rather than target pain as a symptom that signals that something is physically wrong.

Tensions within the pain medicine tradition

In the 1980s, when the authors were at medical school, pain was viewed by clinicians and researchers as more than a hardwired response to a specific stimulus. In 1965 Melzack, a psychologist, and Wall, a physiologist, had introduced the gate control hypothesis of pain (Melzack & Wall, 1965). The gate model suggested that sensory inputs interacted in the spinal cord to help modulate neural transmission and pain sensations. While this ensured the continued focus of pain researchers on neuroscience and the biological processes underlying pain, it also opened the door for psychologists to investigate the effects of attention, memory, mood and learning on pain perception (Meldrum, 2003). In the 1970s, in response to the idea that pain behaviours can be maintained through positive or negative consequences, Fordyce introduced targeted behavioural strategies to manage pain (Fordyce, 1976). The International Association for the Study of Pain was formed in 1973 specifically as an interdisciplinary organization (Bond, Dubner, Jones & Meldrum, 2005). Soon after, Engel published his classic paper on the biopsychosocial model, a reaction to his concerns that the biomedical focus on disease reinforced both reductionism and mind-body dualism (Engel, 1977) while excluding psychological and social factors, and neglecting the patient as a person.

Training influences

The medical school that the authors attended was one of the first to embed Engel's model within the undergraduate curriculum. The programme was designed to humanize medicine. Students worked with patients from their first year of study, communication skills were an essential component of the course, and all medical problems were examined from a biopsychosocial perspective. Stephanie went on to specialize in consultation liaison psychiatry, a sub-specialty in which clinicians work with physicians and surgeons to help broaden their understanding of the psychological and social dimensions of illness. Chris is an anaesthetist, and while his specialty training was very biomedical, his spiritual beliefs helped to broaden his views about illness and patient care, and influenced his perception of what was possible in pain management.

> The year before HIPS was established Chris witnessed a remarkable event at a Christian healing conference. Lynda, a young woman in her twenties, had volunteered to participate in a demonstration of a particular type of healing prayer. Two years earlier she had fallen down a cliff in the mountains while night hiking with a missionary training group. She sustained multiple injuries including fractures in her face and spine, and spent a cold dark night in a ravine with paramedic support arriving in the early hours of the morning. It was not until daylight that the rescue helicopter was able to winch her to safety and transport her to the local hospital. She was discharged from hospital after six days, but went on to develop chronic low back pain and other physical symptoms including fatigue.
>
> A group of around 150 conference delegates observed the session. The process began with the two prayer leaders inviting Lynda to recall the events of the night of the fall. Her story was then followed through to the hospital and subsequent rehabilitation phase. Throughout this healing journey Lynda's deeper emotions were allowed to surface within the context of a supportive environment. Lynda lapsed into a trance-like state as she relived her experiences of the accident and the surrounding circumstances. She was able to recall her shock and fear while lying at the base of the cliff. She had felt angry when a paramedic called her a "whinger" and guilty that

she had fallen in the first place. The fall had occurred in the context of conflict with one of the group leaders. Afterwards she reflected that the trauma had affected her body, mind and spirit.

The prayer brought a sense of peace and warmth into the midst of the relived encounter. The prayer leaders acknowledged God's presence at the time of the accident and throughout the rehabilitation period. They identified both positive and negative spiritual influences that had the potential to amplify whatever was happening at a physical level, and invited Lynda to become aware of and release blocked emotions. Forgiveness played a central role. The result was that Lynda's pain and fatigue disappeared. She reports that her miraculous healing has been sustained over subsequent years (Scott, 2010).

HIPS Foundations

The story described above unfolded during a year of full-time training in pain medicine for Chris at a major Sydney teaching hospital. In that setting there was no opportunity to discuss or even consider pain stories such as Lynda's. When HIPS introduced outpatient clinics the following year in Newcastle, the model of care provided at that Sydney teaching hospital was used as a foundation. This was consistent with a traditional, and in retrospect somewhat dualistic, interpretation of the biopsychosocial model in pain medicine. Patients referred to the service typically underwent a multidisciplinary assessment with a pain medicine specialist, a physiotherapist and either a clinical psychologist or liaison psychiatrist. Subsequent management involved a choice between biomedical attempts to reduce pain on one hand and a cognitive behavioural group pain management programme on the other. The dominant biomedical focus was offered early with the tantalizing, but ultimately unrealistic, promise of sustained pain reduction from that modality. The offer of cognitive behavioural therapy (CBT) came later after the limits of the biomedical approach were reached. A core belief directing the use of CBT, curiously found over time to be untrue, was that chronic pain would never resolve and that the best that could be achieved was for patients to accept it and learn to cope.

In the early years of the service, the annual referral rate was approximately 1000, around 600 procedural interventions were undertaken each year and pharmacological management was the primary focus for many. Although the cognitive behavioural approach was seen at that time as an ideal intervention, there were only limited places available for a group treatment that required eighty hours of contact time. In addition, many patients were resistant to the approach or assessed as not suitable for a group programme. Hence only fifty patients accessed that treatment each year.

> Jenny was a woman in her forties with many years of treatment-resistant, chronic low back pain. Her story illustrates our early problems with this sequential approach to encouraging patients to pursue all biomedical options before moving on to other broader interventions. After several failed surgeries and medication trials she was referred to HIPS for consideration of intrathecal pump implantation (a device infusing opioid medication into the spinal fluid). Multidisciplinary team assessment revealed an articulate and resourceful woman who had persisted with part-time work despite her pain, and who had no signs of a mental health disorder. Despite our offer of a place on the CBT programme, she was determined to persist with biomedical interventions, and in the absence of major psychological contraindications, a morphine pump was inserted. Unfortunately the initial pain reduction achieved with the device was not sustained. Two years later, after the frustration of many side effects and a lack of functional progress she agreed to removal of the device and CBT programme attendance in the preceding weeks. Despite Jenny's anxieties both the programme and pump removal went well. Afterwards, Jenny went on an extended over-seas holiday, medication-free, and from that point began to make significant gains in multiple domains of life. This left us regretting the initial offer of the morphine pump, and wondering why we had not been more insistent in our recommendation of CBT.

Challenges and impetus for change

Despite our best intentions, within two years of the commencement of the pain service, clinicians and administrative staff had identified a number of operational, clinical and systemic problems. There was growing dissatisfaction with the service. Primary care physicians were frustrated with expanding patient waiting lists and a perceived service inaccessibility; patients were increasingly focusing on and demanding the physical interventions offered by the service including intrathecal pumps, nerve blocks and spinal cord stimulators, while avoiding engagement in the CBT and physiotherapy programmes; and despite the attempts to provide a biopsychosocial model of care, pain clinicians were struggling to integrate practice. Conflicts were occurring across specialty lines within the team. Psychologists were sceptical of the biomedical interventions and believed that pain management for patients with persistent pain should focus solely on functional restoration guided by psychology and physiotherapy. The anaesthetists were happy for psychologists and psychiatrists to be involved, but felt that the main allied health role was screening out the "nut cases" or "heartsink" patients so that they could continue their interventions with the more "genuine" cases. One of the anaesthetists had developed a rating system for patients that involved recording a sequence of hearts in a downward arc. The number of hearts corresponded to the degree to which the patient was viewed as difficult or "heartsink." While this was done in jest it reflected a growing sense of frustration and futility that team members were experiencing in treating such complex patients who did not seem to get better. Above all we were worried about treatment outcomes. We had not been collecting extensive outcome data, but our clinical impression was that many patients were happy to return to regular booked appointments for intrathecal pump refills or opioid script renewals, but they were not making functional gains.

In a series of workshops the team attempted to identify and define the issues that were blocking effective team functioning and limiting clinical outcomes. We agreed to focus on several key areas. These included a need to reconceptualize our understanding of the nature of persistent pain, since thinking about pain within the biopsychosocial framework appeared to be maintaining our splitting of the different dimensions. We also decided to look more closely at patient, clinician and systemic resistances to broadening our clinical approach in a more holistic fashion.

The complex nature of pain

Given our training within Western biomedicine it is not surprising that we struggled to see pain in multidimensional, experiential terms. In 1986 the International Association for the Study of Pain (IASP) defined pain as a subjective experience (Merskey & Bogduk, 1994) but despite this acknowledgement the overwhelming majority of medical practitioners still view pain as an object; a marker that something has gone wrong inside the body.

We began to read more broadly around the subject of pain, dipping into anthropological, sociological and philosophical literature, and exploring patients' personal accounts of pain. We particularly admired the writings of Kleinman (1988), Frank (1995), Scarry (1985), Jackson (1994, 2000), Morris (1991, 2001) and Giordano (2008). With the reading came the realization that pain is intersubjective and inextricably linked to meanings and values that are shaped by cultural, personal and situational factors. Our clinical impression of treatment failures began to make more sense to us. Without a shift in model of care to match our expanding view of pain, we could not hope to change patients' experiences.

At the same time we examined the evidence base for current treatment strategies in routine use in the mainstream pain field. This occurred within an international context in the late 1990s of increasing pessimism about the benefits of any biomedical interventions for persistent pain.

The existing evidence base suggests that unimodal biomedical approaches typically produce only modest benefit for a limited time. Problems of tolerance and opioid-induced hyperalgesia (Angst & Clark, 2006, Hutchinson et al., 2007, Ballantyne & Shin, 2008) have major implications for pharmacotherapy. The adverse effect profile of non-steroidal anti-inflammatory drugs limits clinical application (Tielemans, Eikendal, Jansen & van Oijen, 2010). Implanted devices such as intrathecal pumps and spinal cord stimulators have low efficacy and high complication rates (Molloy et al. 2006; Turner, Sears & Loeser, 2007; Kemler, de Vet, Barendse, Van Den Wildenberg & Van Kleef, 2008). Other procedural interventions such as targeted spinal blocks are also limited in degree and duration of benefit (Abdi et al. 2007; Boswell, Colson, Sehgal, Dunbar & Epter, 2007). Furthermore any unimodal use of biomedical strategies runs the risk of distracting the recipient from active management.

The benefits of cognitive behavioural pain management programmes have been more consistently reported in the literature (Flor, Fydrich & Turk, 1992; Guzmán et al., 2001; Morley, Eccleston & Williams, 1999). However a recent systematic review reported only a weak effect on pain intensity, minimal effect on disability, and modest improvement in mood (Eccleston, Williams & Morley, 2009). The authors noted that while the quality of trial design has improved over the years clinical outcomes have not.

At a practical clinical level at HIPS, patients referred often came with high expectations of what might be achieved through biomedicine. Correspondingly there was commonly a reluctance to engage in supported self-management. Certainly many chose not to undertake a high intensity (80 hours duration) cognitive behavioural group intervention. Overall the outcomes at that time were surprisingly poor and we realized that changing our understanding of the nature of pain was only the first step. We were gradually accepting that pain is inseparable from the whole person and that our new model of care and treatment interventions would need to reflect that new understanding.

Patient resistances

One of our initial early concerns was related to how we thought patients would react to our new way of seeing pain. From the beginning we struggled to counter our patients' biomedical focus. While there is evidence that patients are more satisfied with a medical interaction in which they are treated as a whole person (Epstein, 2000; Mead & Bower, 2000) and that patients commonly look outside traditional medical practice to find alternative treatments (Coulter & Willis, 2004), the majority of our patients wanted us to provide a biomedical fix.

There is an extensive medical literature on the concept of somatic fixation. This process, in which patients and physicians inappropriately focus exclusively on the bodily aspects of a complex problem (Van Eijk et al., 1983) is driven by multiple cultural, situational and medical factors. At presentation to our service, most patients were already entangled in the medical merry-go-round.

> Megan is one such patient. She is a woman in her late thirties, with persistent pain in the low back and abdomen, who brought with her a weighty package containing various imaging studies and a folder with pages of neatly documented lists of all medical diagnoses and interventions. She had many mental health problems which preceded the onset of pain and included post-traumatic stress disorder, recurrent depression and multiple suicide attempts. The HIPS team became involved in a tug-of-war about pain causation both

with Megan and other involved medical specialists including two orthopaedic surgeons. Her biological focus, which was shared by the orthopaedic team, had ultimately led to a total of thirteen spinal surgeries. We worked with Megan and her family doctor with the aim of containing her opioid use and balancing the biomedical interventions with psychological support. She disengaged from our service and to this point has not been re-referred. She continues to seek out other medical opinions from time to time and her pain is ongoing.

We all had a tendency to focus on the patient's role in perpetuating the medical focus. It was often easier to label them as somatizers or comment on their abnormal illness behaviour, than it was to acknowledge that a patient's symptoms and behaviour are a product of the health care system, and our dominant biomedical explanatory model for pain. The somatizing label did not make sense for many of our patients who were simply using medical language to communicate with doctors who in turn were only focusing on physical things. Clinicians can easily reinforce a patient's focus on the physical with multiple operations, nerve blocks and investigations.

A further area of patient resistance that the team identified that affected our introduction of a broader approach, was the growing sense of entitlement and autonomy of patients along with the expectation that we were there to give them what they asked for. In part this was encouraged by a medical emphasis on chronic pain as a disease in the nervous system (Siddall & Cousins, 2004) and "pain relief as a fundamental human right" (Cousins, Brennan & Carr, 2004).

> One of our patients was a middle-aged man with chronic low back pain that had proven resistant to oral opioid therapy. He had heard about implanted pumps and was curious to trial that form of therapy. When the assessment process was moving more slowly than he wished he sought help from an advocate who was a member of his church congregation. Pressure was applied with threats of a Ministerial to accelerate the assessment and subsequent implantation phase. This made us more defensive and angry, and we were more likely to label such patients as having a personality disorder or mental health problem.

If we were to adopt a new paradigm, we were increasingly seeing that we needed to educate patients about our new way of looking at things; teach them a different language; show them that we were interested in more than their physical symptoms, and give them very good arguments to convince them that an alternative approach was warranted.

Clinician and team resistances

We held a growing conviction that our patients' behaviours, attitudes and ideas would not change unless we changed our own. In the transformation of our clinical service to a more holistic model of patient care, the biggest challenge has been overcoming the various and multiple clinician resistances.

Boswell and Giordano (2009) have noted that pain medicine as a specialty faces particular challenges in regards to integrating care. The complexity of pain and its unique presentation in individual patients means that clinicians must be flexible and broad thinking, willing to step outside their own specialty areas and function in a trans-disciplinary way. Yet the clinicians on the team had very different backgrounds and training, and struggled to develop a shared language. In contrast, Sullivan (2001) has argued that the very fact that pain medicine as a specialty is heterogeneous gives us permission to mix and match ideas from each discipline and helps us to push and move beyond our traditional boundaries.

In the multidisciplinary clinic, our assessments were sequential; patients would rotate through individual morning sessions with physician, psychologist or psychiatrist and physiotherapist, and then the team met at lunch to further share ideas and formulate a management plan, which was then communicated back to patient and family doctor. On the surface this made us feel that we were all contributing and that the patient's pain was explored multi-dimensionally; but on closer scrutiny, we realized that the clinic structure was simply maintaining our own positions and disciplines in a somewhat rigid way. The anaesthetists and physiotherapists did not have to explore the psychosocial issues because the psychologist would cover that in their time slot. The anaesthetists could rule out serious or harmful physical conditions and feel comfortable that there were no outstanding organic causes for the pain.

While the issues of time pressures, fears of being overwhelmed by patients' emotional problems, and ruling out organic disease were neatly solved, we were a long way from understanding and helping the patient's experience of pain. It did not feel as though our practice was holistic; it had remained firmly split off into different compartments without true integration.

We were able to identify several challenging beliefs held by clinical staff about the nature of pain. Some of these were readily expressed and acknowledged overtly. Others were more hidden and defensive. Outside the team the resistances were even clearer but they were still present in many of us, even though we had specifically chosen to work with people in pain. The more overt examples of labelling patients as "crazy" or "heartsink" were easy to identify and challenge, but there was also a more insidious and subtle process in which the despair, anger, frustration and helplessness of the patients was absorbed and reflected in the emotional stance of clinicians. Some team members dealt with this by deflecting it back on the patients, others had a tendency to withdraw and become detached from both patients and the team, still others would act out their internalized anger by arguing with other team members and for a while there was a noticeable series of mini cross-disciplinary battles. The physiotherapists would often talk about slamming the lid on a can of worms or blocking a crack in the dam wall before the fault widened; they were happy to leave the emotional issues to clinicians with mental health training to explore in more detail. The anaesthetists and rehabilitation physicians were able to retain their sense of control and master their increasing helplessness by narrowing their focus down to the purely biomedical aspects of the presentation. Team members gave multiple overt reasons for shutting down the emotional aspects as soon as they emerged: inadequate skills and knowledge, a lack of time to spend with patients, the feeling that it was not part of their role and the concern that they did not want to change the nature of their relationship with the patient.

Systems resistances

We were often aware of the pressure of time within a busy public hospital system. The burden of waiting lists and the need for patient throughput was always before us. This issue is common to all public hospital pain services across Australia, with an average waiting time of five months (Hogg, Gibson, Helou, Degabriele & Farrell, 2010). In this environment a key part of the challenge of bringing change was to defend the time to stop and think. In some instances our prioritizing of such an approach was recognized and valued by colleagues but more often there was criticism, spoken or unspoken, about the lack of real work taking place.

There was also the challenge, which is ongoing, of communicating our changing views of pain and its management to the clinicians who refer to the service. This has proven particularly difficult in situations when the referrer has the expectation of a more biomedical intervention and our pain clinic view favours limitation of biomedicine and engagement with other aspects of management.

The search for true integration

However much we believed that our patients should be seen in a multi-dimensional way, our biomedical and uni-dimensional training kept directing our patient assessments and it was very hard to formulate their pain problem more broadly. The key issue was that we were not really seeing the person in pain. We all had a tendency to separate out the pain from the person and then dissect that pain into various components, emphasizing the biomedical. While we noted a patient's comorbid psychological issues or social circumstances or current stressors, it was in a mechanistic way.

In retrospect, the start of the solution came when team members came across some academic writings that were not directly targeted at pain per se. Their focus was MindBody medicine. Chris had been consistently reading beyond the constraints of Western biomedicine. A number of authors were particularly influential. Deepak Chopra wrote from the perspective of someone who was raised in an Indian culture and then trained in Western medicine and specialized as an endocrinologist. His response to seeing the limitations of Western medicine was to undertake further training in Ayurvedic medicine and develop an interest in quantum physics. He writes about the MindBody approach and the curious way in which both contemporary science and ancient wisdom traditions speak about the fundamental connectedness of all things and the co-expression of mind and body out of a deeper underlying reality (Chopra, 1989, 1993). Similar themes were evident in Traditional Chinese Medicine and Buddhist teachings. Ainslie Meares (Meares,

1967, 1978), a psychiatrist and early Australian pioneer of MindBody medicine wrote about the power of meditation to restore connection and bring healing from pain and other problems. Ian Gawler, who worked with Meares as part of his own journey of healing from cancer, added an emphasis on nutrition alongside his practice of meditation (Gawler, 1994). For Chris it was challenging to integrate such ideas back into a Christian paradigm which was often interpreted more narrowly. However there were some writers such as Parker J Palmer and Henri Nouwen who were able to embrace similar themes from a Christian perspective (Palmer, 1980, 2004; Nouwen, 1992, 1996).

While these writings were interesting and helped us to move away from the reductionism and mind-body dualism that dominated our clinical practice, we still struggled to apply developing thoughts about personhood to our patients. We felt we needed practical strategies to help us restructure our clinical approach. We found these in the work of Brian Broom, a New Zealand physician and psychotherapist whom Stephanie had met at a psychoanalytic conference in the late 1990s. Broom's writings present a model for understanding the inextricable integration of disease with subjectivity and mind (Broom, 1997, 2007). More importantly they offered practical suggestions for tackling these dimensions in the clinical space. Most of the HIPS clinicians were not particularly interested in theoretical or philosophical discussions about pain. They wanted concrete suggestions about what to do with patients.

In retrospect, two key areas stood out as being particularly useful for the team. The first was Broom's discussion about the importance of attending to language in the patient-clinician encounter (Broom, 2007, pp. 37–51). This is not just because patient language can help to lead the clinician to an understanding of the meanings of illness but because the language of both clinicians and patients influences the way we view the relationships between mind and body. For example, to speak about patients as having minds or bodies, immediately separates those dimensions away from the person as if they were specific objects. In contrast, by using the verb "to be" as in "I am a physical and subjective person", there is less of a tendency to divide the patient's experiences and their physical symptoms. As a team we made a conscious effort to change our language and to incorporate the "I am" usage into both our day-to-day encounters with patients and the HIPS model of care.

The centrality of story for integrated patient centred care

The second area within Broom's writing that was very useful in encouraging us to integrate clinical care, and to see and treat the patient as a person, was his use of story. Stephanie had been following with interest the developing narrative medicine movement and its associated focus on patient-centred care. Writing in the 1980s Kleinman, a psychiatrist and anthropologist, argued that a patient's personal narrative not only reflects the illness experience but can help to order their experiences and communicate specific associated meanings to the physician (1988, p. 49). By listening empathically to the patient's subjective story the physician keeps the interaction patient-centred, and is better able to uncover cultural influences, patient and family explanatory models, symbolic manifestations of symptoms and associated suffering. All of this helps to set the biomedical data in a broad context.

The opening of HIPS in the late 1990s coincided with Rita Charon's more formal attempt to legitimize narrative as a specific component of medical practice with its own competencies and skill base to counterbalance the growing influence of Evidence Based Medicine (Charon, 2001). Charon describes narrative competence as "the ability to receive and honour patients' stories—how to attend to stories, absorb them, respect them, understand their surface and deep meanings, how to enter them, to let them transform their tellers and listeners" (2006, p. 21). She believes that it requires specific training in close reading, empathic listening and reflective writing. Interestingly, Charon was a plenary speaker at the IASP World Congress in Sydney in 2005, giving one of very few non-biologically driven presentations. In her talk she eloquently highlighted the importance of a narrative approach to the person in pain. Chronic pain involves trauma and loss and she believes that telling the story of pain is essential for its healing. Charon invited the audience to complete a narrative writing exercise; a paragraph about one of our pain patients who had particularly moved us. She then demonstrated the art of close reading using her own brief patient paragraph as an example, identifying the associated nihilism, asking us to hear the loss of mobility, independence and confidence in her patient. She asked us whether our own writing included patient losses, the plot of pain or our interior responses to the patient.

For those of us who already appreciated the centrality of the patient story in understanding the pain experience, Charon's ideas were powerful and very moving. However the majority of the very bio-medically focused audience were either bemused or openly sceptical. Morris has examined the multiple challenges and resistances evoked in Western health care professionals by the concept of narrative medicine (Morris, 2008). These range from practical concerns about the lack of time we have to speak to patients to deeper fears that engaging with patients in this way encourages the erosion of professional distance and authority. At the IASP conference, Stephanie overheard three eminent international anaesthetists discussing the unreliability of the patient's story. They believed that multidisciplinary clinics with sequential assessments were a waste of time because they had observed that the patient gave a different story to every clinician, making it impossible to divine the objective truth of the patient's underlying pain diagnosis.

Our attempts to introduce the concept of narrative medicine to the HIPS clinicians were unsuccessful. While all clinicians accepted the benefits of a move to more patient-centred care and the need to explore subjective aspects of the pain experience, it was not entirely clear how this should happen and none of us were prepared to engage in specific activities like close reading or reflective writing about our own illness experiences. Several staff members objected to what they referred to as unnecessarily flowery academic language and labelling. As one physiotherapist said, "If you are talking about the patient's story you should just call it that."

Broom's straightforward and simple discussions of story appealed to this team of busy clinicians. For Broom, "stories" are a way of tapping into the multifactorial dimensions of illness and by listening to them we can help patients make sense of their experiences. By maintaining the focus on story without categorizing the dimensions into specific, discrete diagnoses, whether medical or psychiatric, we can maintain the patient's individuality and uniqueness.

We invited Broom to Australia to lead a number of workshops and seminars for both HIPS team members and interested clinicians outside the hospital system. The workshops were practically focused and highlighted the specific clinical skills necessary to identify the important details of a story, recognize the underlying meanings and themes, and create a warm and supportive clinical space where the patient is comfortable to discuss their ongoing experiences.

HIPS new model of care

In developing a new model of care the challenge lay in improving integration both at the level of the individual and the broader system. After much team discussion of concepts and language, two diagrams (Figures 1a and 1b) emerged to illustrate the "whole person" approach. From this perspective the pain experience was not confined to the body and in fact could point to difficulties with any aspect of personhood (1a). An expanded view of management followed (1b) with the new aspects of story and nutrition added to the various elements of the traditional biologically focused strategy and the thoughts and actions emphasis of cognitive behavioural therapy. Although in reality "story" encompasses all dimensions of the person and their treatment we decided to include it diagrammatically as a component of management to highlight its crucial role within the new model. Significantly biomedicine came to occupy a more humble position in the context of the holistic approach. The focus on the patients' choice of multiple management options invites therapeutic balance but maintains the notion of individuality. Of course management choices are not entirely patient driven. HIPS team members use their expertise to encourage patients to consider particular management options that suit individual clinical situations.

At a systems level, we focused on developing an efficient model of care and the wise use of limited staff resources. Within the redesign process a key task has been to hold the tension between such system

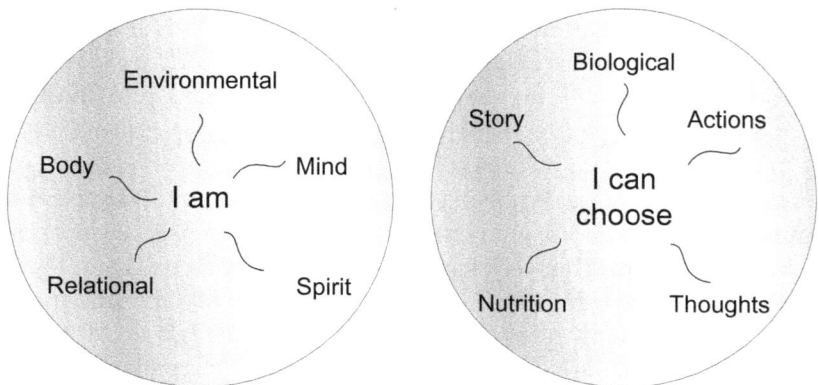

Figure 1a. A whole person model.   Figure 1b. Whole person management.

efficiencies and the need for a truly patient centred, whole person approach (Hayes & Hodson, 2011). The key components of an ideal model of care for patients with persistent pain include multidisciplinary capacity with integrated, holistic practice and consistency of key messages across community, primary and tertiary levels of care. We felt it was particularly important to provide education and feedback to family doctors since they carry the main burden of managing persistent pain in the community.

The new HIPS model addressed both the need for integration between the multiple levels of the health care system (Figure 2) and a more multidimensional approach to each unique patient.

At the tertiary level, specific referral and discharge criteria were developed and patient flow pathways were defined. The first point of face-to-face contact is generally the Understanding Pain seminar, a ninety minute session which provides information about the HIPS model of care, highlighting the multiple dimensions of the pain

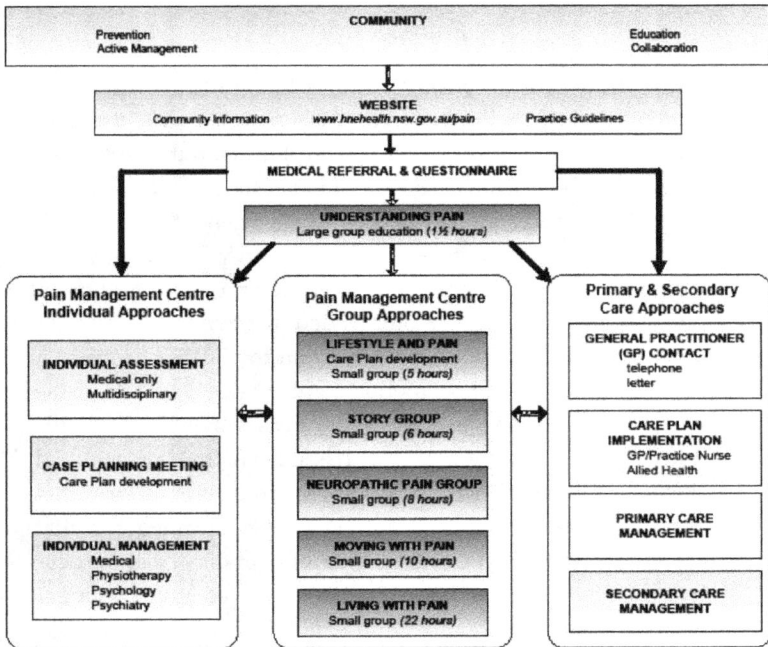

Figure 2: Hunter Integrated Pain Service Model.

experience and informing patients about the range of management choices that are available to them. The Understanding Pain seminar has proven to be an effective waiting list management strategy, and patients and their families are offered a place within one month of referral. Given our extensive geographical catchment area, if patients are unable to travel to the hospital they are sent a DVD of the session to view at home. Multiple short group interventions for patients are then interwoven with individual sessions to target various aspects of pain management. In addition a range of resources are offered to the general community, health professionals outside the hospital and family doctors, by means of a website and other educational material. The availability of a broad range of educational materials and management options has been an important facet of the HIPS model. Patients' pain experiences are unique; many patients with persistent pain will never access tertiary level services, and many patients are not ready or willing to change their views about the nature of their pain. Emma, Anna and Michael are all HIPS patients and their stories illustrate this point well.

Emma's story

Emma's father rang HIPS for advice about his nineteen year old daughter. She had had eighteen months of pelvic pain that had been extensively investigated by gynaecologists, but despite two laparoscopies the doctors had been unable to give her a definitive diagnosis and there had been no improvement in her pain. A general surgeon did not think that the pain was related to the gastrointestinal tract. Emma was booked for an urgent multidisciplinary assessment and we recommended that, while awaiting her appointment, she read some material from the HIPS website that highlights the link between emotional and physical aspects of the pain experience. When she presented for assessment two months later it was with the somewhat surprising news that her pain had resolved. In the website material she had read with interest that physically expressed pain may carry a deeper meaning and that events in the period leading up to onset of pain may be of particular interest. She identified that her pain had started after a younger sibling had been severely injured in a motor vehicle accident. She told us that she had thought about the link and while she did not completely understand it, her pain had resolved within a few days.

There had been one short period of recurrence of pain in the context of some bullying behaviour from a workplace supervisor. This too had resolved when she consciously thought about the links between her increased emotional distress and pain. Emma expressed interest in attending a mindfulness course and was discharged from the HIPS service. At a telephone contact six months later she reported that she remained pain free.

Anna's story

Anna is in her early thirties and has an Aboriginal family background. She was married to a humanities student at the time of her referral to HIPS in 2010. She had difficulties with widespread muscular pain and fatigue from the age of fourteen and had been given diagnoses of fibromyalgia and chronic fatigue syndrome by several medical specialists. After attending the Understanding Pain seminar she chose to progress to a HIPS multidisciplinary assessment. Her appointment was scheduled four months later. During that time it emerged that she had radically changed her diet and had lost six kilograms in weight. She had also independently initiated regular contact with a local counsellor.

At the multidisciplinary assessment she spent much of the time discussing her difficult childhood. Her father was often absent but when present was verbally and physically abusive. She described her mother as a very strong woman who was determined that her children would succeed in the world, but could be scathing when the children made a mistake or failed at a particular task. Just prior to the onset of Anna's illness her father left town after his business closed, her mother went back to work and Anna was left to balance school work with looking after her younger siblings.

Anna was very receptive to the idea that her pain and fatigue were multidimensional and that they might reflect her taking on an increased burden within the family. She was keen to understand her experiences more fully. We offered her a HIPS workbook entitled *Exploring the MindBody in Persistent Pain*. This provides a series of practical exercises that people can work through individually and aims to help patients develop an increased awareness of their inner life. They are encouraged to explore potential links between traumatic life events and changes in health status, and are invited to consider any underlying personality features that might affect their illness experience.

Anna was happy to continue with her nutritional approach and planned to commence a physical programme with a comfortable daily walk and some stretches and exercises. She tapered and ceased her opioid medications since they had not brought much benefit.

Anna was reviewed at HIPS ten months later. She had followed all aspects of the multidimensional plan. She particularly found the MindBody workbook helpful and reported an eighty per cent reduction in pain and fatigue. Given Anna's childhood experiences, cultural background and her own drive to succeed it is not surprising that she accepted and completed all aspects of the HIPS programme without resistance. However most of the patients we see find the idea that pain is multidimensional very confronting and we have to work hard to gradually introduce new concepts.

Michael's story

Michael is a middle aged man who was referred to HIPS with persistent neck pain that had followed a motor vehicle crash fourteen years earlier. At multidisciplinary assessment Michael told us that at the scene he observed that the driver of the other vehicle was under the influence of drugs. Michael became enraged, began to attack the other driver and had to be restrained by onlookers. The question arose as to whether Michael had felt anger like that before and he readily shifted focus back to childhood physical abuse at the hands of an alcoholic father who was now deceased. He was also very angry that after a three year compensation claim process he received only a minimal payout and was forced to accept a disability support pension. No medication trials had worked effectively and he was considering further surgical opinions despite several surgeons already giving him a clear message that surgery was not advisable.

Michael's suggested management plan included biological, psychological and nutritional components. We recommended a three month treatment period with gabapentin, an anticonvulsant medication, to help wind down his sensitized nervous system. This was offered as an alternative to the ineffective combination of anti-inflammatory drugs, codeine and paracetamol that he had been taking. In regard to his nutrition and lifestyle, smoking cessation and reduction in alcohol and refined carbohydrates were recommended. In addition we offered him a place in the Moving with Pain group with the option to progress to the more psychologically focused Living with Pain programme if he wished. We gently explored with him the benefits of tackling the deeper story issues and the associated anger that was firmly entwined with his pain.

Michael refused all suggested treatment options and has been lost to follow up.

The story group

Many of our patients do not initially feel comfortable either sharing their story or exploring with us the underlying meanings or their broader experience of pain. At the point of referral they have typically seen multiple providers. They are angry that the health care system has not met their needs; they have commonly been labelled as "frequent flyers" or "nut cases", and their stories have been dismissed as either not relevant or pointing to a psychiatric diagnosis. They are distressed and feeling a loss of control, and they not unreasonably assume that HIPS staff will treat them the same way.

The Story Group is a key part of HIPS strategy seeking to normalize the exploration of deeper meaning. The group is a four session psychotherapy intervention for eight to ten patients led by two psychiatrists. While we initially planned to offer brief dynamic intensive psychotherapy it quickly became evident that very few patients met our selection criteria. These included psychological-mindedness and a desire to look more closely at the connections between emotions and pain and to delve into pain meanings. However, most of our patients were suspicious of any intervention that they thought might enclose them in a psychological box. To attract a larger number of participants, and in keeping with our views about the importance of story as a means of making sense of the pain experience, we opened the group to everyone, and changed the focus of therapy. The group provides a safe place where patients can share their story, interact and compare their own experiences with others with persistent pain. The therapists' main role is to help the group make sense of their experiences, identify patterns in the stories and make links to underlying emotions that had previously been unrecognized by patients. While we have not yet run enough groups to meaningfully assess outcome data, we have been surprised by our patients' willingness to not only tell their pain stories but at their ability to identify underlying emotions and links with previous traumas. Many patients who were previously very biomedically focused have used the group as a stepping stone to progress to individual psychotherapy work.

Challenges and future directions

The use of an integrated, holistic model of care has led to a gradual reduction in emphasis on biomedicine. While many patients remain guarded about the significance of the broader dimensions of their pain experience and avoid treatment that is not biologically focused, they are given many opportunities to explore other options. The HIPS model of care has evolved dramatically over the past decade in line with our changing views on the nature of persistent pain. Biomedical interventions are no longer considered to be the primary management option. There has been a dramatic reduction in the number of procedural interventions that we offer patients and we no longer implant intrathecal devices or spinal cord stimulators. We are able to offer patients a broad range of multidisciplinary management options and our team functions in a more integrated, trans-disciplinary way. Team members respect and tap into each other's expertise, but feel comfortable working across disciplines.

The focus on the patient story has been the most significant factor in our move towards more holistic and integrated practice. It keeps our practice patient-centred and is a vehicle for tapping into the multiple dimensions of the pain experience. All team members are comfortable with the term "story" and it has become accepted as everybody's business across all disciplines. Our referral questionnaires, management plan summaries and our feedback to family doctors and patients all routinely include a story component. However, learning to listen to and work with patients' stories has not been easy. The initial enthusiasm has been tempered by the need to process the associated anger, distress and frustration that is a core part of the pain experience. We have managed this with regular debriefing sessions and supervision meetings for staff, but we frequently struggle to contain our own and patients' emotions, and it is sometimes tempting to fall back on a more distancing and controlled way of interacting with patients. We also commonly find ourselves editing patients' stories so that they fit specific diagnostic categories or patterns. At times this is appropriate but sometimes it reflects our learned tendency to categorize and simplify the situation. One team member became so enthusiastic about the concept of the patient story that he would look for meaning in all aspects of the patient encounter, get caught in the complexity of the presentation and ignore or minimize biological factors, illustrating a degree of story reductionism. Team meetings provided a good opportunity for members to support each other but also to challenge our departures from the HIPS model and maintain a balanced focus across multiple dimensions.

At a recent team meeting we discussed staff perceptions of how things had changed for HIPS in the past decade and where team members thought we were headed. A consistent picture emerged of a service that had undergone a major transformation. Staff recalled the late 1990s HIPS as chaotic, with a sense of being underfunded and understaffed. The focus on managing biomedical aspects of patients' pain presentations meant that the anaesthetists were under pressure to perform the medical reviews that only they were qualified to complete. Waiting lists expanded quickly which caused distress to patients, family doctors and hospital administrators. Interdisciplinary tensions increased. HIPS administrative staff described spending much of their day fielding complaints, and the non-physician team members felt devalued and unable to use their expertise.

All team members agreed that, while HIPS is still evolving, team functioning, goals and the model of care are now very different. The regular scheduling of team meetings and education and planning days has been an important means of ensuring a culture of collaboration and trust between all team members. Clinical and non-clinical staff understand that their ideas and suggestions will be considered and that team conflicts will be addressed overtly. The change in our working model of pain has ensured that all team members feel valued and have a clearly defined role to play in more person-centred care. In the discussion, staff identified that they now feel more confident in tackling the emotional and affective dimensions of the patient's pain experience, something that all clinicians, apart from the psychologists and psychiatrists, had actively avoided previously. There was also a sense that we have developed a reasonable balance between the needs of our individual patients and the demands of the health care system with its focus on waiting lists and its steady pressure to move patient treatment back to the community. The HIPS website, with its range of resources for patients, allied health practitioners and family doctors, has ensured that patients have the opportunity to apply our model of care to their own pain without a need for our direct intervention.

In the next phase of development we will continue to focus our research on quantifying the impact of our evolving model of care. It has taken us some years to develop a culture of outcome measurement and benchmarking. Our initial resistance to close scrutiny of our clinical work and our deeper fears of systemic change have been overcome by system demands; and a skilled team psychologist who has gently guided us to a point where we now collect outcome data on all aspects of management. This facilitates the ongoing process of adapting our treatment interventions according to clinical and resource effectiveness. As a team we are happy with the position that if any of our interventions are not successful they will be changed. Whatever the future holds, there is a collective determination within the HIPS team to continue to defend the safe spaces in which stories can be told, and in which transformation happens.

References

Abdi, S., Datta, S., Trescot, A. M., Schultz, D. M., Adlaka, R., Atluri, S. L., Smith, H. S. & Manchikanti, L. (2007). Epidural steroids in the management of chronic spinal pain: a systematic review. *Pain Physician, 10(1)*: 185–212.

Angst, M. S. & Clark, J. D. (2006). Opioid-induced hyperalgesia: A qualitative systematic review. *Anesthesiology, 104(3)*: 570–87.

Ballantyne, J. C. & Shin, N. S. (2008). Efficacy of opioids for chronic pain: A review of the evidence. *Clinical Journal of Pain, 24(6)*: 469–78.

Bond, M. R., Dubner, R., Jones, L. E. & Meldrum, M. L. (2005). The history of the IASP: Progress in pain since 1975. In: H. Merskey, J.D. Loeser & R. Dubner. (Eds). *The paths of pain 1975–2005* (pp. 23–32.). Seattle: IASP Press, 2005.

Boswell, M. V., Colson, J. D., Sehgal, N., Dunbar, E. E. & Epter, R. (2007). A systematic review of therapeutic facet joint interventions in chronic spinal pain. *Pain Physician, 10 (1)*: 229–53.

Boswell, M. V. & Giordano, J. (2009). Reflection, analysis and change: The decade of pain control and research and its lessons for the future of pain management. *Pain Physician, 12*: 923–928.

Broom, B. (1997). *Somatic illness and the patient's other story. A practical integrative approach to disease for doctors and psychotherapists.* New York/London: Free Association Books.

Broom, B. (2007). *Meaning-full disease. How personal experience and meanings initiate and maintain physical illness.* London: Karnac.

Charon, R. (2001). Narrative medicine: a model for empathy, reflection, profession and trust. *Journal of the American Medical Association, 286*: 1897–1902.

Charon, R. (2006). Suffering, storytelling and community: an approach to pain treatment from Columbia's program in narrative medicine for pain. In: Flor, H., Kalso, E. and Dostrovsky, J.O. (Eds). *Proceedings of the 11th World Congress on Pain. 19–27* Seattle: IASP Press, 2006.

Chopra, D. (1989). *Quantum healing.* New York: Bantam Books.

Chopra, D. (1993). *Ageless body timeless mind.* New York: Harmony Books.

Coulter, I. D. & Willis, E. M. (2004). The rise and rise of complementary and alternative medicine: a sociological perspective. *Medical Journal of Australia, 180*: 587–589.

Cousins, M. J., Brennan, F. & Carr, D. B. (2004). Pain relief: A fundamental human right. *Pain, 112*: 1–4.

Eccleston, C., Williams, A. C. & Morley, S. (2009). Psychological therapies for the management of chronic pain (excluding headache) in adults. *Cochrane Database Systematic Reviews*, April 15; (2): CD007407.

Engel, G. L. (1977). The need for a new medical model: A challenge for bio-medicine. *Science, 196(4286)*: 129–36.

Epstein, R. M. (2000). The science of patient-centred care. *Journal of Family Practice, 49*: 805–807.

Flor, H., Fydrich, T. & Turk, D. (1992). Efficacy of multidisciplinary pain treatment centres: A meta-analytic review. *Pain, 49*: 221–230.

Fordyce, W. E. (1976). *Behavioural methods for chronic pain and illness.* St. Louis, MO: CV Mosby.

Frank, A. W. (1995). *The wounded storyteller: body, illness and ethics.* Chicago: University of Chicago Press.

Frank, A. W. (2005). Generosity, care and a narrative interest in pain. In: D.B. Carr, J.D. Loeser & D.B. Morris (Eds.) *Narrative, pain and suffering* (pp. 289–300). Seattle, WA: IASP Press, 2005.

Gawler, I. (1994). *You can conquer cancer.* Melbourne: Hill of Content.

Giordano, J. (2008). Pain, depression, brain-mind and healing: the potential complementarity of process and purpose. *The Pain Practitioner, 18 (2)*: 7–12.

Guzmán, J., Esmail, R., Karjalainen, K., Malmivaara, A., Irvin, E. & Bombardier, C. (2001). Multidisciplinary rehabilitation for chronic low back pain: systematic review. *British Medical Journal, 322 (7301)*: 1511–6.

Hayes, C. & Hodson, F. (2011). A whole person approach to persistent pain: from conceptual framework to practical application. *Pain Medicine, 12 (12)*: 1738–1749.

Hogg, M., Gibson, S., Helou, A. & Degabriele, J., Farrell M. J. (2012). Waiting in pain: A systematic investigation into the provision of persistent pain services in Australia. *Medical Journal of Australia, 196 (6)*: 386–90.

Hutchinson, M. R., Bland. S. T., Johnson, K. W., Rice, K. C., Maier, S. F. & Watkins, L. (2007). Opioid-induced glial activation: mechanisms of activation and implications for opioid analgesia, dependence, and reward. *Scientific World Journal, 7*: 98–111.

Jackson, J. E. (1994). The Rashomon approach to dealing with chronic pain. *Social Science & Medicine, 38 (2)*: 823–833.

Jackson, J. E. (2000). *Camp pain: Talking with chronic pain patients*. Philadelphia: University of Pennsylvania Press.

Kemler, M. A., de Vet, H. C., Barendse, G. E., Van Den Wildenberg, F. A. & Van Kleef, M. (2008). Effect of spinal cord stimulation for chronic complex regional pain syndrome Type I: five-year final follow-up of patients in a randomized controlled trial. *Journal of Neurosurgery, 108 (2)*: 292–8.

Kleinman, A. (1988). *The illness narratives*. New York: Basic Books.

Mead, N. & Bower, P. (2000). Patient-centeredness: a conceptual framework and review of the empirical literature. *Social Science & Medicine, 51*: 1087–1110.

Meares, A. (1967). *Relief without drugs*. London: Fontana Books.

Meares, A. (1978). *The wealth within*. Melbourne: Hill of Content.

Meldrum, M. L. (2003). A capsule history of pain management. *Journal of the American Medical Association, 290 (18)*: 2470–2475.

Melzack, R. & Wall, P. D. (1965). Pain mechanisms: A new theory. *Science, 150 (3699)*: 971–9.

Merskey, H. & Bogduk, N. (1994). *Classification of chronic pain*. (2nd ed.), Seattle, WA: IASP Press.

Molloy, A. R., Nicholas, M. K., Asghari, A., Beeston, L., Dehghani, M., Cousins, M. J., Brooker, C. & Tonkin, L. (2006). Does a combination of intensive cognitive-behavioural pain management and a spinal implantable device confer any advantage? A preliminary examination. *Pain Practice, 6 (2)*: 96–103.

Morris, D. B. (1991). *The culture of pain*. Berkely, CA: University of California Press.

Morris, D. B. (2001). Narrative, ethics and pain: Thinking with stories. *Narrative, 9 (1)*: 55–77.

Morris, D. B. (2008). Narrative medicines: Challenges and resistance. *The Permanente Journal, 12 (1)*: 88–96.

Morley, S., Eccleston, C. & Williams A. C. (1999) Systematic review and meta-analysis of randomized controlled trials of cognitive behaviour therapy and behaviour therapy for chronic pain in adults, excluding headache. *Pain, 80*: 1–13.

Nouwen, H. (1992). *The return of the prodigal son*. New York: Doubleday.

Nouwen, H. (1996). *Can you drink the cup?* Notre Dame, IN: Ave Maria Press.

Palmer, P. J. (1980). *The power of paradox*. Notre Dame, IN: Ave Maria Press.

Palmer, P. J. (2004). *A hidden wholeness: The journey towards an undivided life*. San Francisco: Jossey Bass.

Scarry, E. (1985). *The body in pain: The making and unmaking of the world*. New York: Oxford University Press.

Scott, L. (2010). *Lynda: From accident and trauma to healing and wholeness*. Lancaster, UK: Sovereign World.

Siddall, P. J. & Cousins, M. J. (2004). Persistent pain as a disease entity: implications for clinical management. *Anesthesia & Analgesia, 99 (2)*: 510–20.

Sullivan, M. D. (2001). Finding pain between minds and bodies. *Clinical Journal of Pain, 17*: 146–156.

Tielemans, M. M., Eikendal, T., Jansen, J. B. & van Oijen, M. G. (2010). Identification of NSAID users at risk for gastrointestinal complications: A systematic review of current guidelines and consensus agreements. *Drug Safety, 33* (6): 443–53.

Turner, J. A., Sears, J. M. & Loeser, J. D. (2007). Programmable intrathecal opioid delivery systems for chronic non cancer pain: A systematic review of effectiveness and complications. *Clinical Journal of Pain, 23 (2)*: 180–194.

Van Eijk, J., Grol, R., Huygens, F., Meeker, P., Mesker-Niesten, J., van Mierlo, G., Mokink, H. & Smits, A. (1983). The family doctor and the prevention of somatic fixation. *Family Systems Medicine, 1*: 5–15.

CHAPTER EIGHTEEN

Training "troops" for a MindBody revolution

Josie Goulding

The MindBody Healthcare programme at AUT University, Auckland, New Zealand, offers a revolutionary approach to health practice. The need for it springs from the current situation in Western healthcare, in which Cartesian thinking underpins most practice and services. The clinical experience of the open and observant practitioner testifies on a daily basis to the inefficacy and irrelevance of much modern healthcare, which often seems distant from the human experience of illness and suffering of the patient.

The MindBody approach involves a scrutiny of the healthcare philosophies and assumptions that are largely implicit in modern practice, and goes on to challenge and greatly expand them. Theories of mind, body, personhood, relationships, systems, and illness and disease, which emerge from both Cartesian and post-Cartesian philosophical standpoints, are explored. All this is done in very close relationship to everyday clinical practice, which in the process is radically re-appraised and re-focused. The MindBody approach is radical, and extends through and from the classroom to the clinical practice room, and from person to person, and small group to small group.

We weight the programme towards a phenomenological and relational way of thinking, which sits in contrast to the empirical model currently embedded in Western culture and health care practice. MindBody concepts demand a science that supports complexity, interconnectedness, and life that is emergent and relational rather than static and isolated. We are interested in understanding the patient's individual experience of their illness and its origins and meaning, and not just descriptively looking for a formulaic match with what we know about disease already. "Embrace complexity and refuse the sirens of reductionism" (Orange, 2010) could be one of the mottos of the programme.

The shift from a dualistic philosophical position towards a whole person approach stresses the importance of returning to the phenomena of clinical presentation and practice. In this perspective the patients emerge as persons before the practitioner. The phenomena always precede understanding or interpretation. Therefore attention to the patient, and to the relationship between the patient and the clinician, becomes the clinical ground and a starting place for a more dialogic way to hold practice and theory.

This type of practice is demanding, both in its call to view the patient as a whole and as a unique individual, and in its style of interpersonal engagement required to participate in a unique healing journey with each person.

This change in focus, to what is happening for the patient, for the practitioner, and in the relational space, and why it is important, will be the subject of this chapter. Moreover, I will explore the remarkable parallel between my own process, the student's processes, and the processes patients experience when invited to engage in this way. To give some flesh to this, I will share some of my own experience as well as some of the student's stories.

The phenomena of practice: an example

Three students were demonstrating the touch-based techniques they used with their patients. Some fellow students eagerly volunteered to be the recipients, because previous role plays in the class had been almost entirely talk-based. The role play practitioners commented on what they were doing as the play unfolded, and some of the recipients had powerful experiences. During one particular play the therapist commented that he could not feel anything, or, more specifically, he felt an absence over a part of the recipient's body. This was not taken any further in the session.

However the next day in class during a reflective space the patient reported that she had been upset and in a deep emotional process since the role play. The absence comment had been very significant, both metaphorically and physically, and related to an area of personal experience and growth that had been active in her life for a long time. She was able to give the other student practitioner feedback about the experience, telling him what was helpful and distressing about it. She was clear that the practitioner had been astute in what he was experiencing; she was able to invite a more interpersonal engagement from the clinician concerning his responses in the role play, and to say that she would have liked him to make more meaning with her at the time, so that she was not left alone in her upset state. She felt she had gained from the experience, even though she would have liked more from the practitioner at the time he made the comment. He, in turn, was grateful for the feedback, although upset that he had not been aware of his impact on her. By implication he was challenged to think and feel about how he impacts on his patients and how he reflects on interventions with them. This was not a comfortable interaction at some points, but was a powerful learning opportunity for the whole class, which grew out of the students' openness to learning from each other, and giving enough class time to process their experiences.

What can we learn from this?

The practitioner in this role play is primarily a touch practitioner, although he talks with his patients, helping them make sense of their illness. His perception of what was in deficit and negatively affecting the patient was accurately felt through touch. But the meaning of this was not storied between them and an opportunity for creative development of the moment was not taken. This was a splitting in practice, if not in the practitioner's mind. It was also a lesson about slowing down, and paying attention to the impact of his comment, seeing it both as an intervention and a subsequent opportunity to process what was to be learnt and utilized for healing. In other words, what was seen as clinically important needed to include not just the clinical symptom for diagnosis or understanding, but also perception of the patient's reaction and the importance of the interpersonal connection in processing this reaction.

What do we attend to?

Philosophy informs theory, and theory configures what we experience and see in practice. Despite this inescapable reality, most health practitioner education pays scant attention to the theories of knowledge, health, wellness, personhood, body and mind underpinning clinical practice.

For example, the connections between the phenomenology philosophy tradition and psychotherapy development and practice seem obvious and important, and I am interested in why these connections and the phenomenology theorists were omitted from my psychotherapy training. Donna Orange in her recent book *Thinking for Clinicians* (Orange, 2010) recognizes this shortfall in many psychotherapy education programmes in the United States, and asserts the helpfulness for clinicians of such philosophical explorations in providing the grounds for a more critical approach to their practice, and in an ability to support their own thinking when confronted with the forces of a more technologically focused world and health environment.

Kant, Husserl and Heidegger all proposed in their own ways that "philosophical purposes must be satisfied prior to any practice of psychology" (Owen, 2006). I contend that this is not just important for psychology but for all healthcare practice. Currently, most practice defaults to the dominant dualistic philosophical position, which splits mind and body. This split results in a dismissal of much relevant clinical material, and minimizes or negates a suffering person's subjective experience and meaning. The result is a reduction of their experience of humanness, and an alienation from themselves and the practitioner. Additionally, this creates an imbalance in the relative value of ways of knowing, weighting the process in favour of the practitioners' beliefs in their objective observation and clinical knowledge. These effects frequently detract from the health and agency of the patient.

Teaching and practice

In the MindBody programme students experience a teaching method, which is analogous to the clinical practice that we are advocating. It is grounded in a phenomenological, relational, inter-subjective mode of engagement. Moreover, it sits within the humanistic tradition, which Orange (2010) defines in this way:

"The humanistic tradition in Europe includes a set of inclinations ....
(a) a Renaissance/Enlightenment preference for thought over superstition or authority; (b) an aversion to all forms of scientific reductionism or "it all comes down to" thinking; (c) a valuing of solidarity, dialogue and inclusion; and (d) an ongoing interest in what constitutes a good human life" (p. 8).

These elements position the programme and ourselves as teachers, and shape our invitation to students to think about what they do, why they do it, how they are in relationship with their teachers and patients, and what their aims are in their practice. For practitioners of all disciplines, the programme is a clear alternative to the culturally dominant Cartesian model.

Phenomenology as a way forward

Husserl and Heidegger, two prominent twentieth century critics of Descartes, were the early primary contributors to the branch of philosophy called phenomenology (Orange, 2010; Loewenthal, 2011; Stolorow, 2011). Heidegger developed Husserl's ideas, blending phenomenology extensively with constructs such as hermeneutics, contextualization and existentialism in exploring and conceptualizing our being-in-the-world (Loewenthal, 2011; Stolorow, 2011).

A contemporary, critical reading of Heidegger and the work of other phenomenologists, certainly can influence and expand our understanding of the task at hand, or even what is possible, when a patient seeks help. This contributes to our view of what is useful clinically and informs our practice in important ways; particularly by focusing on and being deeply interested in what actually presents to us; or, as van Manen (1990) suggests, "interested in the human world 'as we find it' in all its variegated aspects" (p. 20). Phenomenology encourages a move away from judgement towards understanding. By doing this it opposes reductionism, and demands that we see our patients as whole persons relationally connected to the past, present, and future, the places and people around them, and the meanings that these experiences are embedded in and engender.

This deep phenomenological interest is not just in what is easily accessible by conscious reflection on the part of the patient and therapist, but, from its inception with Husserl, phenomenology has been "centrally concerned with the structures that pre-reflectively organise conscious experience .... and in particular those that give meaning to emotional and relational experiences" (Loewenthal, 2011). In order to access pre-reflective and therefore non verbalised experience in the therapeutic relationship we need to turn our attention to our own experiences. Lowenthal (2011) asserts that gaining understanding "involves us in attending to our experience in all its richness, mind, body, actions, without censure, as a primary source of information for our practice rather than using theory as our immediate reference point". Traditionally, health practitioners are often taught to focus solely on the patient as the source of clinical information and then to move to theory for understanding. This shift in focus, from attending solely to the patient's experience, to including the experience that is generated in the space between the practitioner and the patient, and to the experience of the practitioner while in relationship with the patient, is a challenging dimension for many.

What is more, clinicians often feel there are inherent dangers in clinical information that feels more subjective than objective, and thus trying to decide between subjectivity and objectivity often becomes a concern. Merleau-Ponty, another phenomenologist, is helpful in thinking about this. He introduces ideas that break down a range of dichotomies that we think of as discrete domains of experience; for example, inside and outside, conscious and unconscious (Zeddies, 2000; Merleau-Ponty 2005). In doing so he highlights the difficulties of radical subjectivism and objectivism (yet another dichotomy) and invites us to consider inter-subjectivity as a way forward. Entering the inter-subjective space means we are open to noticing the effect that patients have on us and we have on them as part of understanding who they are, who we are together, and how we might work together therapeutically. Of course, such a process also challenges practitioners to notice who they are, and the chapters of this book are ample testimony to how this is worked out in practice.

The phenomenological stance, along with other principles, lead to the following emphases in developing the students' growth into Mind-Body practice:

1. Humans are complex and are situated in their own personal developmental history.
2. Humans are relational and meanings-orientated, therefore health and illness involve these dimensions of human being.

3. Theory is secondary to experience.
4. The body, both the patient's and the practitioner's, is central to experience and needs to be closely attended to.
5. Attending to the patient's experience by holding open a space for thinking and relational engagement with the patient, and being open to what is emerging inter-subjectively between the patient and the practitioner, allows meanings to emerge, and develops a possible space for healing. Careful attention to this process allows the practitioner not to foreclose by imposing their solution on the patient.
6. Meaning and interpretation are always secondary to experience or the phenomena. However, meaning is also constitutive of experience. In practical terms, the meaning of the patient's illness is both part of the pre-reflective phenomena and available for emergence, development and change in the relational space with the practitioner. "Nothing can be grasped that the relationship does not allow" (Stern, 1991, pp. 70–71, as quoted in Zeddies (2000)).
7. Psychodynamically-informed understandings of interpersonal communication, relational skills and formulation are the background we draw on to hold the interpersonal space.

The positioning of the clinical relationship as central to clinical practice and the teaching programme is based on its importance in understanding the patient's particular suffering or situation, and for its role in the healing process. In understanding relationship, we follow the philosopher Levinas, introducing students to the ideal that presupposes all practitioners can and do have an ethical responsibility to be present, that is, relationally available, and clinically interested in the particularity and otherness of the patient they are working with. This is based in Levinas' understanding of the other; the other who is never able to be fully understood, and therefore not subjugated to our pre-knowing or our belief that we can fully understand the other (Morgan, 2011).

It is therefore an engaged-with or "a responding relationship rather than a knowing relationship" (Donna Orange, Wellington Workshop, 2012) that we are asking the students to consider in theory and practice. In this way we are inviting the students to adopt a posture of not knowing in the relational interaction, which is contrary to what most practitioners expect of themselves in practice. This is a challenge to the idea of what constitutes the expert health practitioner in a traditional

Western model. It does not mean that the practitioner gives up their traditional expertise, but instead that they can function in both ways seamlessly or interchangeably in the same time and space.

This focus on meaning and relationship often takes the students on a new journey. The patient with their disease is not an object to be discovered or uncovered, but a subject to be engaged with in a mutually effecting relationship. This call to relational practice uncovers both personal and existential issues that can trigger huge relief, because often there is recognition of what is already known by the student or patient. It can also generate personal challenges, even "fear and dread" (Lowenthal, 2011). Adopting the MindBody approach, with its challenge to knowledge, clinical practice and personal identity, can stretch a student's capacity to manage interpersonal anxiety. This is the most difficult aspect of training and many find a need to engage in personal psychotherapy to process their experience.

The beginning: my personal journey

The challenge of teaching MindBody Healthcare, which came to me unexpectedly, sparked a re-evaluation of issues that I had chosen to relegate to the past, or gloss over and separate from.

My first qualification was in nursing, working mainly in the community with families as a public health nurse (health visitor in the UK) and in sexual health, HIV testing and treatment, and more general issues of sexuality. Whilst I enjoyed this work, I became frustrated, finding that my physical and (sometimes) socially-orientated interventions were often inadequate in the face of the psychosocial issues facing the patients. I was trained to assess the patient's problems and come up with solutions or treatments. Whilst in principle we were supposed to work collaboratively with the patient to formulate solutions, we were ill-prepared to do this. Rather, the training was more orientated towards encouraging patient compliance to accepted solutions.

More than this, I felt frustrated with the results of my referrals to specialists to address the psychological difficulties that I felt were components of so many of the more difficult and distressing patient's situations. Such referrals led to assessment and diagnosis and, at best, some interventions, many of which had the same deficits as those I deployed and left me in the community with a patient in whom very little change occurred. It seemed that diagnosis took precedence over the capacity to work compassionately with the person as a whole.

I felt inadequate to address this felt gap, and embarked upon psychotherapy training. My difficulties then came in trying to integrate nursing and psychotherapy ways of working and this had mixed results. There were some extremely positive outcomes, but mostly these were achieved with a struggle and also contributed to some painful relational difficulties in the workplace. Finally I withdrew into a much safer environment: private psychotherapy practice and teaching in a psychotherapy programme. This allowed me to escape my workplace discomforts and challenges, and, from the haven of psychotherapy practice, to project my bad feelings on to the medicalized health system.

However, my interest in the overlap between physical and psychological health and the connectivity of the mind and body led me to writing a Master's thesis on the therapist's experience of their body during the therapeutic relationship, using hermeneutic phenomenology as my research methodology. Connecting the epistemological and ontological underpinnings of thought and theory allowed me to begin a more thoughtful personal positioning with regard to my practice and what I taught.

"That which we dread"

Then the opportunity to teach in the MindBody programme appeared. Even though theoretically and experientially my practice had led me in the MindBody direction, and I had continued to work with clients presenting with physical symptoms, I did not have a strong grounding in theory relevant to mind and body integration. These anxieties about not being up to the task of teaching, not having my ideas integrated for myself, and being dependent on Brian Broom, my co-teacher, for the content of the programme, were echoes of my earlier history.

Sometimes I reacted by being rigid about what I thought I knew, and, at the same time, feeling de-skilled. These elements interfered with my teaching, particularly with the earlier cohorts of students. Reflecting on this, I recognized two linked issues. The first was the very different teaching styles of nursing and psychotherapy training, which reflect elements perpetuating the MindBody splits in the health sector generally. More importantly, I now realize that I was still holding mind and body as mutually effecting but separate spheres, rather than a central unity from which mindful and bodied experiences could be perceived. The felt experience was difficult to put into words, but, in retrospect, it is clearly related to the paradigm shift that we ask students to make while still working in the dominant health culture. For me, there was a feeling that if I was teaching non-psychotherapists I needed to provide the kind of teaching that I had experienced in my nursing training. This involved the imparting of knowledge, and knowledge that was presented as truth. This type of teaching relates to a more positivist paradigm, typical of healthcare settings that are dominated by the medical model. This was also what some of the students expected.

My anxiety even extended to the teaching of the more philosophical components of the programme, which one might think would naturally lend themselves to a more interactional and phenomenological approach. While a phenomenological approach was at the heart of what we were introducing, my anxiety about being taken seriously in mainstream health settings led to feeling I should present a more technologically-focused teaching programme. Any move away from a technology-based emphasis is counter-cultural, not just for the medical system, but for Western society generally.

For me, fear occupied the gap I experienced between a phenomenological and relational approach to working with students and a positivist, more quantitative scientific approach. Loewenthal (2011) names this fear as "that which we dread," a fear we hold individually and culturally when entering unknown or "transitional spaces".

I realize now that in moving away from healthcare towards psychotherapy I had held this split within myself. As I began to teach on the MindBody programme, my initial inability to think about this more deeply or coherently was related to anxiety spiked by my return from the safe haven of psychotherapy to mainstream physical health settings, as represented by the students (from many different health care disciplines) and Brian (an active physician as well as a psychotherapist). I was, in effect, back in the arena I had previously found distressing.

Whilst much of my tension could be construed as residues of past struggles with the healthcare system, it remained a lively current issue working and teaching in a MindBody way in a university health faculty where the positivist paradigm and medical model is dominant on many levels. This dominance is seen in research grant funding favouring measurement approaches, and in some departments where teaching can be overly linked with conforming to registration board or professional certification requirements, or professional orthodoxies around a practitioner's relationship with evidence-based practice. It is expressed in inter-departmental conflicts, particularly in the context of the drive towards interdisciplinary teaching. Examples of this include the role and place of diagnostic tools in assessment and a reliance on more formulaic teaching of interpersonal skills and therapies such as Motivational Interviewing and Cognitive Behavioural Therapy. It is not that these modes of practice are not useful but that they are applied in a blanket non-person-centred fashion.

Teaching in the MindBody programme was more challenging than teaching on the psychotherapy programme because in the latter I could immerse myself in that particular orthodoxy. To join, at the expense of my own knowing, or to reject those who did not agree with me, had previously seemed the only options. Adopting a relational, phenomenological way of working as a MindBody teacher would not allow me to maintain this split unchallenged. While the retreat to psychotherapy or to theory can be helpful to create some framework and parameters and reduce the fear of chaotic experience, it can also restrict the creative aspects of engaging with what emerges interpersonally. In short, such retreat shuts down the possibilities for other ways of bringing these positions together.

The second part of the struggle was to both hold my individual experience and to stay relationally connected, which has a lot to do with my role in my family of origin. I have needed to address the way I hold responsibility with regard to others, and more particularly how I hold involvement, empathy and separation; and this has been a focus in my personal therapy and supervision over the years. This is a personal and professional task and, I believe, a continually emergent and useful process that allows me to address issues that are triggered within the teaching context.

This fundamental paradigm shift, created by positioning myself in the interpersonal and subjectively focused ("being with" rather than "doing to") field of practice creates challenges to do with the change in the clinician's personal experience of working with patients, and the cost of holding this different position systemically. This change can be distressing for students, confronted with their own anxieties triggered in interpersonal encounters. In order to teach this way of being in practice we must model the phenomenological and relational focus in the teaching. At the beginning I knew this in theory, but was struggling to find the capacity in myself with any consistency.

Challenges in the classroom

Reflecting on what it is really like in the class room, two challenges stand out. The students come from a wide range of backgrounds, both personal and professional. In terms of the health sector they come from both the traditional medical and the complementary or alternative ends of health practice, and so the range of material that can present in the context of the programme is vast. This diversity has been part of the joy of working with the students, but it means the students can have very different learning needs and, like me, the learning challenges they face are both personal and professional. The variety is a valuable aspect of developing and teaching on this programme, as we discover ways to bring the MindBody approach into clinical practice across the spectrum. We are clear that we do not want the students to abandon their previous professional identities and modalities of practice, unless of course the MindBody approach makes these redundant. We do however wish to make them more thoughtful about the way they work and encourage them to adopt a meanings-orientated and interpersonally focused way of working and thinking.

The second challenge for me was finding my way back to what I know about; that is, working in the interpersonal space, in the face of both my anxieties and those of the students.

The diversity in the classroom

All the students on our programme are experienced health practitioners of some mode of practice. They are adult, informed and competent in their own discipline. This makes a huge difference in introducing new material. What we are aiming for is to broaden their capacity to really listen to, or, perhaps more accurately, experience their patients (however they receive their information, for example through touch, talk, or vision) and then use the information to explore relationally what is being presented, from the perspective of the whole person of the patient, always in the context of their own disciplines.

As described above, a part of my initial defence in facing this challenge was to go to theory in a split off way. In the class room, however, theory is both wanted and not wanted by the students. For the most part the students already believe that there is a false dichotomy in separating the mind and the body. This may arise from previous reading, or intuitive and experiential knowing from their own lives and practice. What they most want is to know how to change their practice to work in a MindBody way. What they are looking for theoretically is to deepen their understanding, partially to convince other health professionals with whom they work that these MindBody ideas are valid; indeed their versions of my own struggle. A few come to have their way of working as MindBody practitioners legitimized, and this can be difficult if it does not seem to us that they are actually working in a MindBody way.

I do not want to minimize the theoretical component of the programme however. While theory can be used defensively, it can also be rejected defensively. It is clearly important to the deepening of the student's reflexive practice. It does not replace the attention to experience, but gives the practitioner a broader range of material to draw on in attending to their patient's experience as well as their own. Being able to provide a strong theoretical and reflective base for practice is something that contributes to a professional rigour that most health professionals hold as important, particularly if they are going to change what they do. The process of developing differing and new concepts of rigour is, I believe, part of the programme's role and its challenge to the students.

Staying with the phenomenological

The race to "what do I do?" has an intensity born of practice anxiety; of wanting to be able to offer something immediate to the patient, who is often pressing them for something tangible. Trying to come to this from the extensive and often complex literature applicable to the MindBody approach can lead to what can feel like an essential gap between the theories used to explain aspects of MindBody unity and how to address this understanding in everyday health practice.

The exploration with the students of staying close to the experience in the relationship, discerning how to listen to the patient and how to use this experience in the inter-subjective space, is a very different learning to that which they are accustomed; a clinical paradigm shift. It requires the practitioner to bring their genuine presence, not just their expertise, to the engagement. Interestingly this includes the complementary health practitioners, many of whom are actually taught from a positivist paradigm, as their various disciplines try to gain status and legitimacy in the medically dominated health industry.

For some students their difficulties reflect their starting places. Psychotherapists are more daunted by the actuality of bodies and illness, and the physical nature of illness presentations; and are biased towards providing psychological explanations or diagnoses for the patient's difficulties. Non-psychotherapists and body practitioners are more daunted by the talking components and the attention to the emotional and relational material in the patient's presentation. The students face re-evaluation of what their involvement could be, and overcoming the feeling that their area of least knowledge cannot be dismissed simply as not being within their "scope of practice," and facing the fact that such dismissal is, often enough, better seen as a splitting off of what they were not prepared to listen to.

Whether they are the anxieties of body or mind practitioners, they lead to distancing behaviours in the practitioners. Yet all practitioners are there because they recognize patients in their practices that they want to be able to be more effective with. Often they are also faced with work environments that do not support a more personalized integrative type of practice, but believe that specialization and technological approaches are the most effective for all patients both time-wise and financially.

Practice anxiety

Taking a more phenomenological and existential approach to working with the patient faces clinicians with the gap and the fear of the transitional space by inviting, accepting and embracing the experience of not-knowing through deep reflection on what is. Instead of racing to match symptoms with solutions, the invitation is to prolong the not knowing by engaging in mutual exploration with the patient. It heightens a practitioner's own anxiety and involves having to sit with unknowing in a way that most health practitioners try to avoid by being experts in their field of knowledge. This anxiety is more commonly recognized and understood by the psychotherapists in the class, but knowledge does not offer protection from the experiences that are generated in the confluence of the individual contributions to interpersonal relationship and the cultural context. My own difficulties in the classroom exemplify this.

A practitioner may retreat because of the intensity of transferential and projective processes, particularly in patients who find that the pain that the illness is expressing, or pointing to, is easier to tolerate as illness than knowing about it in clear conscious awareness. For the practitioner to continue to maintain that an illness is, for example, a storied expression of internal experience, when it manifests as a known, medical condition which has drug treatments available, can feel too much responsibility to hold; even when the medical treatments are not offering the patient illness resolution or relief. This loss of confidence in the importance of staying with the exploration of phenomena and meaning is also often a reaction to the patient's pressure for someone to know the answer or provide the cure.

Students often present situations of this sort in the class for discussion and we ask them to role play the situations. This can be exposing, but also creates huge learning opportunities. The role plays are both an opportunity for the student to experience first-hand what it is like to experiment with working this way in a supportive environment, and the opportunity to ask them to notice their own experiences as they work in the role play. Personal responses are something that many health professionals are not expected to pay attention to, or even discouraged from noticing and exploring. An example of a typical patient experience of the type described above came with one of the first patients in our current MindBody research project.

> Joe presented with chronic treatment-resistant urticaria and severe angiodema. He agreed to enter a research progamme in which he was offered ten sessions of MindBody-orientated psychotherapy. He and the therapist quite quickly identified that his difficulties were related to unexpressed interpersonal conflict. He did not seem particularly interested in exploring the underlying causes of his difficulty. He set about rectifying his situation by expressing his conflicts to those around him, and this worked well initially, significantly reducing his symptoms. During the therapy any relapses in symptoms related to times where he had difficulty identifying his conflicts, and symptoms resolved when he expressed his feelings. His wife however was not happy with his change in behaviour; she was stressed by his more confrontational responses,

and complained to both Joe and the researchers about this. Joe did not engage in further reflection. He expressed gratitude about being listened to by an understanding person but reverted to his pre-therapy accommodation to interpersonal conflict. The marital relationship settled down and the symptoms returned.

Unpacking the complexity of this vignette and the therapist's experience of it is very like what happens in the classroom. We would focus on the therapist's (student's) experience of the role play therapy, and what meaning or understandings can be drawn from observations by the protagonists in the role play. Using the example of Joe, the question arises whether Joe chose a flight from a confrontation with his family that did not work for him, and perhaps to some degree reinforced his relational fears. It appeared the couple were happier with the sometimes life-threatening symptoms than with addressing the anxiety-provoking and possibly painful implications of the underlying meaning of the illness and the relational issues. Further, the example shows that even though the patient was able to use, in this case, a talking approach to connect the occurrence of his symptoms to their emotional triggers, he was not willing or perhaps able to process the underlying meanings of his reactions.

Reflection with the therapist about his felt responses to Joe would help the therapist reflect on their work together. The degree to which Joe's symptoms represent a very difficult emotional experience for him can only be guessed at, from the severity of what was a potentially life threatening condition. A different solution not involving illness might require a life-changing relational focus. Where does this leave the therapist and the patient? This case is an example of how difficult it can be to dwell together with what is not consciously available to the patient, in this case the patient's relational anxieties. What could be felt by the therapist, for example, the patient's anger and fear, may have precluded the patient's interest in himself and his relationships; including the therapy relationship. What can be learnt from reflecting on this? As a MindBody group we can play with and explore what is available to us from the encounter and where this may have gone if more time was available. Incidentally it also shows the difficulty of having a set time frame of individual therapy; in this case a time limitation set by the research project, but often enough a reality of much healthcare practice. Interestingly the couple continue to seek allergy and food intolerance solutions to the problem with no success.

The use of play in learning and interpersonal practice

The notion of play helps to describe and engender the type of relational space that facilitates meaning-making in both the teaching context and the therapeutic relationship. Loewenthal's (2011) emphasis on working relationally, attempting to generate this potential space for play, with its attendant ethic of unknowing, is very helpful. Synthesizing material from Donald Winnicott and other sources, he clearly articulates that this unknowing is not a disavowal of knowledge per se, but the unknowable quality of what will take place between us as we open ourselves to encounter each other. He delineates three issues that are at the heart of teaching, learning and practising the difficulties of working in a Mind-Body way.

1. First, relatedness includes a need for separateness in order that play can occur.

This could be seen as a very Western concept particularly if we equate separateness with autonomy. Certainly Loewenthal (2011) puts forward ideas on autonomy and heteronomy and their relative privileging. Personally I think that while heteronomy may be defined as the opposite of autonomy, the definitions of both derive from Western thinking. Coming from New Zealand (a country where indigenous challenges to the Western privileging of autonomy as the goal of developmental maturity is a controversial topic), entertaining alternative possibilities requires just the kind of not knowing, and commitment to engagement in dialogue, that we are discussing as a goal of relational practice. This raises the question whether there may be other states of being, not centred in autonomy, that allow and foster interpersonal play.

Play, as it is meant here, presupposes the achievement of the states of experiencing one's self as both the doer and the observer. This requires the capacity to recognize a differentiation between our internal state and the outside world. The model does suggest that the interactive capacities of reflective functioning[1], mentalization[2] and the use of potential space,[3] and therefore being able to experience, think about our experience, and to make meaning of it, are necessary for play. It relies on being able to understand that other people have a MindBody that is subject to experience, and are able to step back and think about the experience and attribute meaning to it. It also incorporates the capacity to understand that the other person may have a different meaning to one's own. It is in the interaction between the two persons' subjectivities that creativity is potent.

It would be wrong to see this as a fixed capacity, but rather one that is varyingly available to us depending on our history and situational anxiety. However, Lowenthal's implication is that the type of separateness described above is a prerequisite for the type of interpersonal play that leads to the emergent stories between clinician and patient that allow healing to occur.

The acceptance that there are experiences different from our own, and which may either be unknowable personally or change our own experience of how we understand ourselves, can be deeply disturbing and leads to Lowenthal's second point.

2. Entering the relational space of "unknowing" can lead to a reminder of that which we dread.

Lowenthal refers to two such reminders. Firstly, past adverse relational experience can be transferred or projected onto the current clinical situation preventing us from being surprised by the fresh and original nature of the encounter. Secondly, rather than stimulating creativity and life we may be brought close to more extreme fears of relational loss or annihilation, and fears of death(s); for example, the death of thinking.

We often feel interpersonal anxiety when confronted with the difference or separateness of another person, particularly if the difference has a potentially negative or conflicted meaning. This is heightened by the power dynamics inherent in certain relationships and our cultural settings. At their most extreme these fears are of relational loss or annihilation, and a common response is to defend ourselves by either subjugating ourselves or dominating the other interpersonally. Either of the above defensive positions moves away from complementarity in the relationship, and limit the possibility of experiencing the difference as valuable and therefore creating a potential space for play (Benjamin, 2004).

For me it was necessary not to collapse into my previous experience with colleagues in the health sector, but stay with the tension in the classroom to enable a more creative solution to emerge. It meant paying attention to my responses in the class process and disciplining myself to find personal processing space outside the classroom. I had other experiences in the class where I did not feel restricted by these issues, and the contrast made it easier to see when I was becoming restricted.

As my awareness increased I could much more easily use the new experiences to respond from. In the programme, my easy relationship with my co-teacher also meant that this could be explored and modelled to some extent in the classroom, because we were able to disagree, debate and play with ideas in the class. It was what we were asking the students to do, and this invitation to join in this play allowed students to experiment. I am not intending to dismiss the inherent power dynamics in the classroom, particularly students' desires to conform in order to be accepted, liked, and to pass the course; but I believe we at least partially address this by encouraging an atmosphere where it can occur, and by giving ample space to thinking about what is generated by reflecting on each session as a group.

Predictably, we found that students are most challenged by the interpersonal components of the programme and the personal challenges of their own histories. The material demands of the participant reader (here I mean reader of text in the broadest hermeneutic sense, in other words, reader of theory, patient presentation, story, and body) to engage with a genuine openness to learning, and this cannot help but stimulate self-reflection. However "reflection has to come from desire" (Symington, 2011). This is perhaps both the easiest and hardest part of the teacher student engagement in the class room. Students who want a more formulaic answer to what to do, or who do not want to open themselves to change and challenge, will struggle. The invitation to this type of reflective practice is not able to be picked up by all students. Most students however take up the challenge and many of the previous chapters attest to this. The feedback from many students has been that one of the most powerful benefits of the programme has been the way they have made use of the programme to engage in a personal developmental process in much the same way that I have been describing for myself.

Engagement of this type requires us to open ourselves to the impact of the other, whether that is in the form of knowledge, relationship, or change of world view. Letting myself be affected by what I am learning or by the patient I am working with (learning from) is a risky business. Entering the unknown in this way holds the possibility of growth, creativity and learning, as well as loss, crisis and hurt (Casement, 1991; Loewenthal, 2011; Symington, 2011). It is not long before students are asking about personal therapy and supervision, which are very important in developing MindBody practice.

> One of the students (a body therapist) comes to mind here. During the MindBody programme she was referred a patient who had an abuse history. Contact with this patient impacted the practitioner in a way that she had not previously allowed. The patient had a very strong emotional effect on the therapist and she decided to seek supervision to process this and to be able to stay present to the patient during the sessions. This was a new approach, and was a painful and sometimes confusing experience for her. Some short time later the patient had a very strong emotional release during a session. She became aware that, in being able to stay present to her own emotional responses during the therapy, without distancing herself from what was happening, she allowed the patient in turn to connect to his emotional material in a way that he had not been able to do previously. It was both difficult and demanding because it required the student to make herself open and available to what was present for the client (very distressing experiences) and between them. Ultimately this was a very rewarding for both the therapist and the patient.

Our difficulties in staying with the model

None of us need to be convinced of the MindBody non-dualistic approach; that is why we are involved in the programme. In practice, however, internalized dualism keeps surfacing; perhaps not unlike internalized racisim, where the cultural knowing sets up conflict with experiential knowing or restricts the horizons (Gadamer, 1989) that frame our view of what is possible. I often find myself caught in statements and ideas that reflect dualistic thinking, and also fears of what might be evoked if I move outside not just what is known, but what is acceptable in the teaching of health practice.

An example of this is the inclusion of spirituality in the programme. We were tentative around how and when to introduce this aspect of practice, theory, understanding and meaning-making into the programme. In my experience spirituality is an area that is treated with great anxiety in the health care setting. It is usually left to the patient to initiate any spiritual discussion and, given it is not introduced to the patient as relevant to health (except as information collected on admission to hospital in case the patient needs a priest or minister), why would they? Spirituality is nominally included in many models of holistic practice but most practitioners are wary of it in case they are seen as pushing it onto the patient. In the teaching of holistic models it is often left to a mention in passing. New Zealand is a predominantly secular country where organized religion does not play a major role in most people's lives, therefore spirituality is not overt in the dominant culture and is often underrated in its importance. For those who do choose to have a religious practice it is therefore very significant, and spiritual beliefs are integral to and strong in Maori and Pacifica cultures represented in New Zealand. Spiritual practice is often attended to publicly in these culturally sanctioned ways. However, spirituality in its broadest sense would seem to be important to many of us, yet, it is treated as though it does not play a role in the meaning people make of their life experiences, including illness. This stance deletes a whole realm of human experience from the consulting room.

In teaching the first cohort of students we left the exploration of spirituality until near the end of the second year of the programme. The students were quite vocal in their criticism of this late insertion. Why, they wondered, had we left this topic important to both them and their patients until the end of the programme. They were right. It was fear of the very things we were purporting to challenge them about that had me so reticent. This combined with the sense that I had to have spirituality sorted out in my own mind and heart before introducing it to the class. Of course this was nonsense. This idea of the classroom as an arena of play, not a platform for the naming of truth, is part of what I have been articulating. The students value the opportunity to explore their own spiritual beliefs and the role these have in their work. They value the significance and space given in the programme to a patient's spiritual beliefs, and the acknowledgment that these can be given attention like other domains of patient experience and belief.

My fear that the students will somehow leave with wrong ideas has been a challenge to me, and I realize that to a large degree this is a fear of professional judgement from my own profession; psychotherapy. More specifically the fear was that I was disseminating professional knowledge outside the profession to groups that do not have extensive psychotherapeutic training and that somehow this would come back to bite me. The grandiosity of this is somewhat embarrassing; however it has freed me significantly to be able to admit it. I have gained enormous respect for what the students have been able to do with the experiences and opportunities the programme has provided for them. Hearing of their clinical work and the poignant interpersonal moments, which have led to change and healing for their patients, and the students themselves, has freed me from these fears and inspired me to want these opportunities to be more widely available.

We now come to Loewenthal's third issue.

3. Consideration of that which resists symbolisation, but which may hold open possibility through the play of language.

This concept captures a lot of the theoretical underpinnings that we teach to in the programme. Clearly in the above statement there is a privileging of mental symbolizing. In working with patients who are using their bodies as their primary expression or symbolization of their pain or suffering this is an important consideration. It is also an area of debate in the class room. What about touch, looking, and experiencing in healing? As a psychotherapist, language is my focus or window. The students are keen to debate its place, and I have felt experientially challenged by them.

There was much that I could not have articulated about my experiences early in the programme. The understandings I have mentioned most fully in this chapter, which were the most easily available through my reflective processes, were the unconscious impacts of the previous work-related trauma. What was much less easy to access was the impact of my early developmental experiences that contributed to the traumatic nature of the work experiences and the depth of my fears. As a psychotherapist I have participated in a good deal of therapy at different times but most recently over the past six years I have been in twice weekly therapy. This has helped me to consciously know more about what is behind my responses. Differing experiences and relationships allow me access to different parts of myself at different times, and in this respect the MindBody programme has been a gift. There is not a "once and for all knowing of myself".

I do not think healing happens by the process of symbolization alone. However, in the process of healing, symbolization allows a more conscious involvement with one's own life and the meaning we make of it; a sense of "owning one's own soul" (Krystal, 1988). This is not the anxious grasp of "controlling through knowing" that I was struggling with, but an owning that can allow a more empathic engagement with oneself and at best can allow more choice and responsiveness. Perhaps it is my bias but I resonate with Socrates: "the unexamined life is not worth living."

In conclusion, the reflection that teaching on this programme has afforded me has challenged me to be more conscious of the basic principles behind my practice rather than the particular knowledge that I bring to it. More than that it has challenged me to revaluate my relationship with that knowledge and how I use it. Even though the relational psychodynamic type of psychotherapy that I am grounded in holds the principles I am discussing, the personal confrontation with myself, in this teaching process, has deepened my understanding and personal commitment to the phenomenological as the starting point for my practice and teaching.

References

Bram, A. D., Gabbard, G.O. (2001). Potential space and reflective functioning; Towards conceptual clarification and prelininary clinical implications. *International Journal of Psychoanalysis*. 82: 685–699.

Casement, P. (1991). *On learning from the patient*. New York: Guilford Press.

Gadamer, H. G. (1989). *Truth and method*. New York: Crossroad.

Krystal, H. (1988). *Integration and self-healing*. Hillsdale NJ: The Analytic Press.

Loewenthal, D. (2011). *Post-existentialism and the psychological therapies: Towards a therapy without foundations*. London: Karnac.

Merleau-Ponty, M. (2005). *Phenomenology of perception*. London, New York: Routledge.

Morgan, M. L. (2011). *The Cambridge introduction to Emmanuel Levinas*. Cambridge: Cambridge University Press.

Orange, D. (2010). *Thinking for clinicians: Philosophical resources for contemporary psychoanalysis and the humanistic psychotherapies*. New York: Routledge.

Owen, I. R. (2006). *Psychotherapy and phenomenology: On Freud, Husserl and Heidegger*. New York, Lincoln, Shanghai:, iUniverse Inc.

Stolorow, R. D. (2011). *World, affectivity, trauma: Heidegger and post-Cartesian psychoanalysis*. New York, Routledge.

Symington, N. (2011). World Dreaming—6th World Congress for Psychotherapy, Sydney.

Zeddies, T. J. (2000). Within, outside, and in between: The relational unconscious. *Psychoanalytic Psychology* 17: 467–487.

Notes

1. Reflective functioning as defined by Bram and Gabbard, (2001).
   The term emerges from ego psychology and attachment theory and describes capacities and attributes of an individual mind as follows

   1. the ability to understand one's own and others behaviours in terms of mental states (thoughts, feelings, motivations)
   2. an appreciation and recognition that such perceived states are subjective, fallible, malleable and based on but one range of possible perspectives.

2. Mentalization is often used interchangeably with this term however Bram and Gabbard (2001) suggest that it is a narrower term in that while it is developmentally achieved through the caregiver-child relationship it functions intrapsychically, is circumscribed to representations of mental states and their implication for interpersonal functioning and is based in procedural memory.
3. Potential Space as defined by Bram and Gabbard, (2001).

   1. originates in the caregiver-child relationship.
   2. involves playing with ideas and symbolic thought.

   They quote Winnicott in describing it as the psychological experience that is located between fantasy and reality and between one's inner experience and the external world. He states that potential space plays a key role in the development and differentiation of the self and because it is the basis for play, creativity, empathy and other factors that lend richness to human experience and relatedness. Ogden (1992) adds that above all potential space is viewed as a state of "coming into being", a sense of aliveness that is an experience significant in itself, thereby transcending its role as developmental impetus ... that is to say, in potential space one is able to think in terms of meanings and play with them, all with some (at least pre-conscious) awareness that it is one's self that is creating such meaning, albeit relevant and real from a personal standpoint, it is not the same as objective reality.

INDEX

For Product Safety Concerns and Information please contact our EU
representative GPSR@taylorandfrancis.com
Taylor & Francis Verlag GmbH, Kaufingerstraße 24, 80331 München, Germany